WRECK

Editor: Susan Musgrave
Cover art: Tania Wolk
Book and cover design: Tania Wolk, Third Wolf Studio
Printed and bound in Canada at Friesens, Altona, MB

The publisher gratefully acknowledges the support of Creative Saskatchewan, the Canada Council for the Arts and SK Arts.

Library and Archives Canada Cataloguing in Publication

Title: Wreck : a very anxious memoir / Kelley Jo Burke.
Names: Burke, Kelley Jo, author.
Identifiers: Canadiana (print) 20210155647 | Canadiana (ebook) 20210155884 |
ISBN 9781989274446 (softcover) | ISBN 9781989274453 (PDF)
Subjects: LCSH: Burke, Kelley Jo. | CSH: Dramatists, Canadian (English)—Biography. |
CSH: Authors, Canadian (English)—Biography. |
LCSH: Anxiety—Patients—Canada—Biography. |
LCGFT: Autobiographies.
Classification: LCC PS8603.U73755 Z46 2021 | DDC C812/.54—dc23

radiant press

Box 33128 Cathedral PO
Regina, SK S4T 7X2
info@radiantpress.ca
radiantpress.ca

For Eric, always.

And for Teen, of course

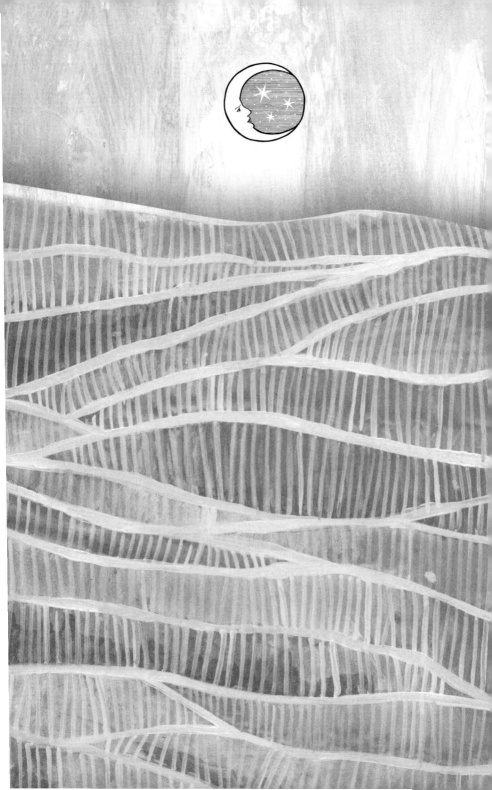

WRECK

a very anxious memoir

Kelley Jo Burke

The author is deeply grateful
for the assistance of the Saskatchewan Arts Board.

Thanks also to Radiant Press, and in particular,
to developmental editor Susan Musgrave,
for her invaluable feedback.

contents

About the Author

You know those memoirs that people write after they've chatted everything over with those concerned, and made sure everybody's good with it and they just want the writer to feel free to speak their whole truth?

This is not that.

Wish it was. I have a freakish memory, which starts when I was nine months old. It is scattered and tattered, but there's lots of it; my bio-hard drive runneth over. I long to dump my whole truth out in the world, make it a thing that exists, has weight and veracity. I think I`d run better.

But my family doesn't have those chats. We have chats where I run memory past them and get told it is shit I just made up. Which kind of makes the floor go out from under my feet. Then I hyperventilate. Get the tingly feeling around my lips, the left chest squeeze. Realize that this isn't a panic attack, but the big one, and I am finally, genuinely dying.

So. Kind of want to avoid that conversation.

Also, there is a real possibility that some of this **is**... shit I just made up.

I am a liar. A good one. Most of my family is. We pride ourselves on it. We are bullshitters. Grifters. Cons. Tale-tellers. Guilders of lilies—and punch-lines. Editors of inconvenient truths. Omitters of inconvenient details. Because, we like to tell ourselves, we can; we are smarter than every chump we hustle.

We have whoppers for all occasions: The speeding ticket. The border tariff. The rule that's for other people. Serves them right for being a mark. Serves them right for charging too much. One born every minute and base is the slave that pays.

That could be you, gentle reader.

Except.

When I was in college, I lived at home, and did not go to the University of Manitoba which was basically next door and where my father taught—but to the smaller University of Winnipeg, downtown—where I was less likely to be greeted as Professor Burke's daughter—as in "You're Jim Burke's girl? But he's such a nice man?"

I took the family car to school whenever I could get it—it was more than an hour by bus. I parked in the only free space on campus—the faculty lot. There were always a few empty spots. I learned which profs were on sabbatical, rode their bikes, had DUI-ed again and were being driven in by their generally younger second wives (former grad students—it was the 80's). Parking anywhere but the faculty lot was difficult and very expensive downtown, and I was practically staff—I was an editor for the school paper. I was far more in the right than the other people who shouldn't be parking there.

The university didn't see it that way. They hired students to patrol the lot. I learned this halfway up the escalator. A handsome young Kenyan I think, maybe Ghanaian, caught me and told me I was in a professor's spot. My lie was instantaneous and gorgeous:

"I know I am. (Full commanding settler magnificent enunciation affronted voice) I'm Professor Burke. Would you like to come with me to my office, and have that confirmed?"

He looked doubtful for a moment, as well he should have, and studied my very young, pigtail-framed face. But the smile that followed was stunning. "I have come to this country, and am trying to learn how to know good from bad all over again. I have to believe that someone who looks so sweet and innocent could not lie...so I will believe you now."

Either he did believe me, and my place in Hell is guaranteed, rock solid, unavoidable, or he knew I was lying, and, if so, well-played sir, well-played.

I can't remember what I said next because it is covered in sticky shame and will not load into recall. I do remember starting my coast up the escalator, exultant, fighting the impulse to queen-wave to the masses. I couldn't wait to get home and tell my family about my stone-cold, ball-bearing, magnificently successful lie. Anticipating their pride in my performance was coursing through my veins like China White.

Except.

The man's smile. He had crossed a universe really, made a trip that a girl from the right end of town could not begin to fathom, and come to this cold, utterly alien place, and gotten ... my lie. And he turned it into a moment to learn trust again.

Stepping off the escalator, I knew two things:

1) Good people did not do what I had done, and despite the family habit, I still wanted to think of myself as a good person.

2) I had a problem.

Thank god I come from a long line of drunks. On both sides — not my parents, but trust me, there's sots a plenty sleeping it off on the family tree. Addiction is who we are and how we expect the world to be, and if addiction be not now, yet it will come, and with it comes the syntax of addiction, all ready to coin the experience and dictate the response, i.e. I had a <u>problem</u>. For addicts, be they drunks, junkies, chimneys, starvers, bingers, lardasses, fuck-it-if-it-breathers or in my case, compulsive liars, having a problem goes two ways: cold turkey or a slow road to the abyss (been there, seen that, did not want the t-shirt). So I told that turkey to strip down and jump in the freezer. In short, I quit lying. Completely.

Well. Almost completely.

So, I'm a compulsive liar. Who wants tell her truth. And has a huge problem telling her truth. Because I'll be called a liar.

At this point, I assume your temptation is to bail.[1]

I get it. I'm with you.

Except.

---

1. Particularly considering this is the first of many footnotes you will encounter in this book. It is sort of a tic with me. I have a lot of tics and this is far from the most annoying.

You know how ex-smokers are the most virulent non-smokers? Well, I'm an ex-liar, and that makes me the asshole stomping around, sniffing the air, screeching "Is someone lying in here? This is a non-lying house. I catch one of you lighting up a lie, and I'm gonna make you eat an entire lie-tray worth of lie-butts!"

The hardest hardcore truth you're going to get is from a recovering liar. There may not be much of it, but what there is, is choice.

So that's something.

The Whales 1996

I stumble over the rocks. Tide's out. Something I should have known, would have known if this were still home. I can hear the lash and rustle of the water much farther away than I'd hoped. And it is so dark.

Be careful, honey.

"Ssssh, Teen. I have to pay attention," I tell my dead grandmother, who has taken to murmuring in my left ear.

The Nubble lighthouse sits across the narrow strait, flood-lit for the tourists. It looks like a movie star ready for its close-up. The shape is right, the keeper's place the platonic ideal of a house with its colonial door and shutter-bracketed windows, but the new floods make it a garish hologram of itself. "Hi. I'm not a lighthouse, but I play one on TV ..."

Only the light proper, a white cylinder capped with a black bowler is itself still. Plain. Sturdy as a Greek column. Red eye held by the cap blinking in soft, firm Ons and Offs. As trustworthy as most things are not.

I watch the stars and stripes flapping on the pole beside the light, the wind from the southeast now, with threads of fog beginning to obscure the somewhat excessive to my now-Canadian eye-pattern of the flag. By midnight the fog'll be thick as cream and I won't be able to find my way back to the cottage at all. Hurry up.

The flag flapping? At night? The American flag is never left to fly at night. My grandfather must be terribly far gone if the lighthouse service is leaving the Nubble flag up, and he's not raised hell with them ... or the mayor ... or the cops. But then my grandfather'd been cut off his 911 services for abuse of privilege.

My urge is to storm over the water and take the flag down. Fold it properly, crisply cornered. Careful to never let it touch ground.

"*It ought to be burned, honey,*" Teen's upstate Massachusetts accent is sepia-coloured, a tintype of a voice.

"I know."

"*It would rather be burned than go on when it has been disrespected like that. Our flag is too proud. And we love it too much.*"

"Tough love, Teen." But what else did you ever know?

I've had dreams, since early, three, maybe two years old, of being able to walk on water. On a bright and breeze-curled sea, I am pretty sure, at least in dreams, that I can catch toe on crest, push off, and launch myself from wave to wave. Catch the next, and never sink. I wake each time, thinking "that could work." So the impulse to stride across the tiny strait dividing the island from the cape and pull down the flag is not a wish but an intention.

It is that kind of night. It has to be.

But no. I will write a letter about the flag to the local paper and sign Teen's name. Let the obits guy figure it out.

Best to get on with it.

I have as many of the whale figurines in my coat pocket as I dared snatch before I left the cottage.

I cooked my grandfather dinner. (Oh god, the dishes, grey fur pelts on each. I'd watched him eat his usual meal of banana and milk, cursorily rinse and replace the bowl and spoon, and this was the result, a cupboard of dishes that not only greeted the user, but asked if she'd like to watch the dancing at the local fungal festival.

How long had it been like this, and why in Christ didn't it kill him? The food I made was awful, the steak frost-burned from at least two years in the freezer, and the creamed corn, the only veg left in the house, well, was creamed corn. But he ate it, without complaint. Which kind of slayed me.

As I watched him gum the mess I'd produced, I quivered with impatience. I needed to get to the water. The old man stumped over to his La-Z-Boy that was his home, bed, and, I very much feared, his john these days. I considered lacing his coffee with Chivas, but didn't dare. Cataract surgery brought one sharp eye back into use in his ruined face, and, when alert, he didn't miss a trick. So I had to wait for the eye, I want to call it beady but it wasn't. It was mistrustful, the eye of a toddler whose treat was snatched by a passing mongrel, angry and on the verge of tears, what a way to spend a century. I waited for the eye to close. And then I grabbed my trench coat.

"I'm going for a walk to the Nubble," I'd said.

Stopped at the bookcase by the door, where a dozen of Teen's whale figurines lived. Tried to be mouse still. Mouse silent. Grabbed five from the dusty shelf. Heard him stir. Cut my losses and all but scuttled under the front door, thinking the whole while "Thank god the .45's not under his chair anymore."

It was months after my grandmother's death for the cops to seize all the old man's guns (there were thirty-six by my last count). He had to use one criminally, brandish it at someone in a not I-am-well-within-my-brandishing-rights sort of way. Then they could seize it … at which point he would get another from the drawer or window sill or sugar tin, the places you would normally expect there to be a firearm, and put it under his chair, in easy reach, locked, loaded and ready to be aimed at the neighbour, the letter carrier, or any number of "summer people" of dubious shade and intention. Which would lead to another gun seized … and another … and … and … and ….

"Your grandfather," said the sheriff of York Beach, Maine, in one of his many phone calls to me, "is one of our more colourful characters."

The day before, almost as soon as I'd arrived, I'd gone around the cottage to make sure they'd not missed the revolver in the utility drawer (gone), the derringer in Teen's bedside table (gone), the Luger the old man kept for shooting the starlings that sat on the power line and shat acid on his car. That one was in the bird feed box on the deck last I checked. Gone. Did he pull the Luger on someone? Did he hear a starling's trilling laugh as he, shaking, peering out his one good eye, tried to aim?

Large buck knives and coshes took up sentry duty where the guns used to be—how he must have fumed as he was forced to set these inferior weapons where serious heat ought to be. The rifles were all still down cellar, but he didn't keep them loaded; they were for shooting animals, not people. And besides. They wouldn't fit under the La-z-Boy.

In a year, after he dies, I will come back to the cottage and try to clean out the remaining weapons, and the endless ammo. The sheriff's office will tell me to turn the bullets in to them—they will use them for target practice. I wonder what kind of practice they'll do with the shot for what looks like an elephant gun. No matter. I load up the ordnance, go to turn it all in.

The look on the desk clerk's face behind the bullet proof glass—because while relentlessly quaint, York Beach, Maine is still in the United States of America—as she watches me waddle in, bent by two grocery bags and my trench coat clinking with bullets—cartridge and pellet, .22 and .44, in boxes and bags and jars, and some hundred or so simply clattering like loose change in my pockets, is worth the effort.

"I called. They said to give this stuff to you."

She points at the arched pass-through indentation where the glass meets the metal counter. I start with the boxes of bullets small enough to fit through; I move on to the Miracle Whip jars, the jumbo zip-locks, tip and pour and pull handfuls from my pockets. A downpour of bullets pings and clatters under the gate, the metal din prodigious. We lock eyes, waiting out the rain. In the silence that follows the last bullet's fall, she says, "You'd be Mr. Adam's granddaughter."

Ayuh.[2]

But that's a year and a bit in the future. This is me on the rocks before my grandfather died. This is the night of Teen's whales.

Everyone, including her grandchildren, called my grandmother, Ernestine Adams, Teen. And Teen collected whales. Figurines, carvings, glasses, prints, a gape-mouthed iron bottle-opener, a cutting board used mostly for cracking lobster claws. She painted them on the pottery her husband shaped, and wore scarves patterned in them over ripple-permed hair, and pinned them to her Sunday-going-to-meeting jackets.

They seemed an odd fit for her. She was born in Westminster, Massachusetts, a couple of hours from the sea. There she lived most of her life tiny, dry, and frightened. Of everything. Of air. Of lightning. And horses. And ice and falling and drowning and cars and used Kleenex and lawn mowers and tractors and swings and cellars and polio and the diseases displaced people bring from away, and in fact *other* people generally, not just foreigners, but, you know, Catholics. They have such *large* families. And don't let's get started on the Jews, though they do know how to look after their money, and you have to respect that.

And the ocean. She was terrified of the ocean. But she loved it more than she feared it. And she kept the whales all over her cottage to celebrate that love that was greater than any fear. And that's why I have to get her to the ocean. Somehow.

So I have stumbled through the low brush that grows between our cottage and the rocks and am now standing on high and dry upper boulders, reviewing my haul from the Great Whale Heist.

---

2. This is a southern Maine expression, which technically means "Yes", but actually means more like "Obviously," "I can't believe we're having this conversation" and "Were you dropped on your head as a child?" Variations include "Y'aaaah" with the "ah" drawn out, which is kinder and includes an invitation to go on; "Yuh, yuh, yuh, yuh, yuh..." spoken as a staccato breath out ("So it goes." "It is as one would expect"), and "Yhuh!" as a sudden intake of breath ("I was right, of course." or less frequently, "Dear god in heaven, you were right").

There's a green wax Sperm Whale marked by my teething, three decades and change past. A nicely rounded one of smoky yellow glass—a right whale perhaps. A ceramic orca, lately of a west coast gift shop, that's going to be a little shocked to find itself in the North Atlantic. A carved wooden creature of some south sea descent. And a pilot whale, black enameled clay, grinning a toothy smile. At least the pilot belongs in the water around the Nubble. I remember spying their black backs curving past the lobster buoys.

I find a steady perch, wind up and throw the orca. Hear it break on the rocks below. Damn. I want it in the water. This whole ritual won't work unless I get the whale *in* the water. I need to climb farther down, to the black, shining rocks, the ones slick with kelp, the ones Teen said *never* to go on. Death by crushed skull and pelvis, if not death by drowning, wave-smacked against assassin rocks. But Death—certainly. She could see it.

But I need to go there if I'm to give the right whale a better shot at freedom than its not-really-a-whale-but-an-orca sister.

Oh honey, no. Please. It scares me so to even think it.

And I see Teen now, almost, in a moment's red lighthouse glow, her cord and bone hands clenched, eyes squeezed against her vision.

Stumble-slide further down—the rocks are dry yet crumble of desiccated crab claws and gull shit, no high-water slime. I throw the right whale harder, and hear a tumble ...*plop* this time. Better. But quite possibly between the lower rocks, and so trapped, doomed to stay there, tumbled to sea glass. That's not going to help Teen.

Fumbling for the sperm whale, I move a little closer to the water. Slip on wet weed, catch myself before I tail-bone into a fall from which I am not likely to rise. Pay with barnacle cuts all over my palms. I'm going to fall in, sure as hell. I am where I no longer belong, doing this daft thing, in the dark. Not a soul knows I'm in the state, except an octogenarian who is barred by law from calling emergency services. And even if rescue came, what would I say?

"I was freeing a very few of the dozens of whales my grandmother collected. Because I didn't free her. And when she got sick, her husband of fifty-plus years, a man who is not happy unless armed and dangerous, took a look at the bill for one day in the hospital and said the hell with that, and made them stick her, frightened and gasping, in an ambulance and bring her home. And it killed her. The same day. He killed her. So I was throwing cretaceous collectibles into the sea. It seems the thing to do."

Death by sea battering doesn't sound too bad compared to that conversation.

Look down at the next rock. Sea moss and snails clearly clinging, the snap and bubble of life waiting for the tide to return.

No. You mustn't.

The sperm whale is now three waxy chunks of sperm whale and my supply is running low. But I am going to do this thing. I will pace my steps by the Nubble's steady gleam. Half-crawl a little further, bleed a little more, until I can set at least one whale, the pilot-- swimming. And tell that whale to take Teen with her, to the lighthouse and beyond, to the open ocean, wide and swelling, where Teen's heart will come to slow roll-thud like the sea, her fear resolve into wrack and foam and finally wash away.

It is not a wish, but an intention.

Take care, honey. Oh. Take care.

"I'm trying, Teen," I mutter, and throw the pilot in.

I Was Born ... 1961

On a gladiola farm. Nobody believes this. One of the problems with being someone known to occasionally refine the truth is that when you deliver a pearl like "I was born on a gladiola farm" no one believes it ever saw the inside of an oyster.

But the tall stalks of flowers, striking, without fragility or scent, one of the few flowers suitable for the restrained tone of Protestant New England funerals, could have given evidence, if they'd still stood in the early '60s. The farm was in Westminster, Massachusetts, where my ancestors' bones have held the better locations in the town graveyard for almost 300 years. My house, which once belonged to my great-great aunt, stood between my grandfather's and my great-grandfather's on a short gravel road off Main Street—and the road carried my mother's family name, Adams.

There was a functioning blacksmith shop where my great-grand-father still mended tools. A cider press that produced a juice that would make all others pure disappointment for the rest of my life. A saw mill, a sugar shack, a wheel and kiln. And a loom. There'd been chickens and horses and oxen and cows and a goat, though they too were gone, by my time. And there were fields once given over in part to gladioli, but also vegetables, blueberries, and stands of corn.

From birth to three years old, my world was our houses and barns and fields and brook, which I had the run of, moving from one building to the other, scooped and swung, held and tossed by my greats and grands and especially by Teen. Steadily watched but also private when I chose. As each adult assumed the other had me, I could make my toddling way to a corner of my grandparents' share of the land, where there was a stand of pines, clearly hand-planted by one prudent ancestor or another, whose trunks grew so close together that by 1963 only a very small child could creep into the fortress they created. The ground between the trees was never anything but a brown, crackling carpet of needle sweetness. The sunlight could send its searching rays in all day and never find me.

As much as self-sufficiency is admired in the family—*you don't pay nobody to do nothing you can do yourself*—I wasn't strictly speaking *born* there on Adams Street. That event took place in Gardner, north of Westminster, as my hometown was too small for its own hospital and my parents too educated and modern for a birth at home.

So I am born. My mother, Ruth Burke, nee Adams, is whacked full of "Twilight Sleep," a mixture of morphine and deadly nightshade used during labour in 1961. This is getting us off on the wrong foot. Because she is not whacked enough. The morphine is to cut pain. The nightshade to create near coma and amnesia. But she is highly resistant to all narcotics, and so is tripping balls while in agony, thrashing and straining at her restraints. She keeps telling the nurses that it's not a baby, it's a monkey that will come out of her—the Cuban Missile Crisis has just wrapped so the effects of radiation and images of Bikini Atoll post-nuclear testing babies—hairy monkey horrors with eyes where nose should be and teeth, oh everywhere and every direction, all horrible—are in the news.

Certainly there'd been a blast seven months before when my mother's pre-marital pregnancy was announced, my parents' parents each mushrooming up according to his or her own class, culture and addictions. The cloud seen in some cases from five or six degrees of cousinhood away. And the fallout always falling out.

First there'd been a quick panicked call to Dad's mother. Jimmy Burke must have been badly off his game because he didn't hear his three aunts, there for the weekly canasta session, as they picked up three of his mother's beautiful, heavy and, in some cases, rhinestone-encrusted extensions. He blurted out, "Ruth's pregnant. We got married." and heard his mother's gasp met in sisterly, practiced, Sweet Adeline harmony, three times over.

I don't know what my mother's parents said. Dad was never able to turn that one, telling the *Adams* about future me and my parents' quick and unattended wedding, into an anecdote. All I know is that my mom was expected to acquire a moneyed husband. Why else was she sent to Bates College to study with the scions of Pepsi-Cola and Chase Manhattan Bank? My father, Irish white trash that he was, made that impossible. And my grandpa hated him for it. Flat out. New England hard. And it never passed.

Now, as I come into the world, my new baby skin beginning to dry and chill, and no hand placing itself between it and the sandpaper air, I am learning that this new life will be, in a number of ways, precarious. My mother, exhausted by her violent fight against the drugs, is wailing about the certainty of my having a monkey's tail. After the horrors of attending to a twilight birth, nurse, I imagine, is thinking hard about slapping mother instead of babe, so she's not stepping in. An older hand, a doctor's, firm, disinterested but serving the purpose, lifts me up and slaps me, old school, because I've been born with morphine and deadly nightshade coursing through my brand new veins, and we baby junkies need a little kick start.

But then. But then. Someone wraps me up, and holds me. Another nurse maybe? I close my tiny mouth, which has not been crying, only gaping, shut my eyes, and breathe.

I believe it happened this way, because it will ever be the shape of my luck: to find comfort only a moment or two later than is good for the development of a stable disposition; press against another's heart, ease the aching mouth, close my eyes and *breathe*. Like breathing's something you only get on Sundays when you're very very good.

Getting In 2017

When you're an artist who relies on grants to survive, there are only two kinds of envelopes that arrive with the funding agency's return address on the corner: the thick one and the thin one. The thick one means that your grant has been approved. The thin one means that you are a failure, and the part before where you called yourself an artist is embarrassing and a mistake; you are wasting your life; no one likes you, and you should definitely take that job at 7-Eleven.

I got the thick envelope. I'd been funded to go home for a writing retreat. My real home. Not Westminster where I was born. Not Winnipeg where I was raised. My grandmother's cottage in York Beach, Maine. I could not believe that they went for it.

I'd been staring at pictures of the inside of the cottage for a couple of years. Now and then. Off and on. Not *at all* like an internet stalker up all hours clicking on photo after photo of someone who is *so* not her boyfriend. I stumbled on the cottage website while surfing for pictures of the Nubble and realized that the neighbour to whom my mother sold, had sold it again, and the new owner was using it as a rental property. I hadn't been in the house since 1998 after my grandfather's death, when I went to pack up the whales, the only thing I asked Teen to leave me. From that day to this, I had not been inside. As I ran my eyes over the pictures of the modest two bedroom interior with its glorious ocean and lighthouse view, my breath caught, and tears started.

I have a recurring nightmare about walking through the cottage and knowing that I'm not *allowed* to be there. That *they* will be back any moment. That *they* are going to catch me. And that I have to make them understand that the whole break-and-enter thing doesn't apply to me, because this is my home.

In the dream, it's always night, because I guess that's when you commit crimes. The living room is dimly lit, not by the bright pedestrian wired-in stuff my grandparents installed when the cottage was winterized, but 1960s lights, sometimes old electric, sometimes burning oil, though I don't remember kerosene lamps being used except once, in a storm. More importantly, the dim light is augmented by the Lincoln stove, which is back where, according to my childhood, it should be. Where nothing else ever should have been. Great black box housing rainbow flames from the burning of salt-crusted driftwood and rope. Offering an embrace to a small body shivering from the umpteenth after-beach shower. Inside that embrace there could be no harm, and one might live forever.

I dream-walk through, feeling like a thief but intent on stealing only the right to be there. Through the kitchen, where the Nubble's lamp winks at my break-in, to my grandmother's bedroom. On the bureau sits her blue and white potpourri jar, full of dried rose petals. I put a handful in the pewter bowl beside, pour warm water over, and release the dead sweet into the living world. And then climb under the white candlewick bedspread and sleep, confident gulls will wake me ....

Except my alarm does. And I am lying panicked in my bed in Regina, about as far from an ocean as one can be. It is the night-morning of a prairie winter, and I have no idea—not where I am or who I am—but *when* I am. Then I remember that the cottage is sold. And I will never have enough money to buy it back. So I can't go in. *Ever again.* And that's a stone on my chest, crushing.

I first felt that stone crush when I was eight and got news that my beagle, Penny, was dead. As I held out my empty arms, shuddering and sobbing until I started to hallucinate, some quite cool part of me, observing the hysteria, understood that it was pointless. It wasn't a negotiation. It was math. The world minus one eczemic, and so child-biting, and so euthanized beagle equalled little Kelley shit out of luck. I would never ever hold my dog again.

In just such a mathematical way was I out of luck and reduced to dreams since the day my mother sold my grandmother's cottage.

But then I found the rent-by-owner posting, and that beagle sprang up from the dead. "I have credit cards. I can call a taxi, a plane, a train, whatever. I can give them money. And *they* will let me in," my brain sizzled. It would be the beginning of a great feminist, mid-80s movie. To the strains of a Marianne Faithfull song, I would jump away from the desk. Slip past my sleeping husband. Wish my three kids all the best and *run*, pushing my Mastercard beyond the limits of budget or decency, until I was where I was supposed to have been all along. Images of us on my grandmother's porch (I feel the beagle would be with me at this point), well past the point of sanity or term of my rental, screaming (and baying) our resistance to forceful removal by the York Beach police, coursed through my adrenaline-soaked brain.

However, the husband would have to wake sometime. The kids might have questions about me blowing their college fund on a life by the sea with a zombie dog. So I looked at the pictures online. And tried to deal with the thought that I could resurrect that dog any time I wanted. If I wasn't ... who and where and when I was.

Then I thought to apply for the grant. I was writing something about the week I went back to try to deal with my grandfather, after my grandmother's death. I wrote a cheeky application, making it sound like giving me money to go to my grandma's house was a cutting edge thing to do. And then tried not to think about it.

Until the thick one came. I held it. Shook and hugged it. Stood very still and with a queer light in my eye, said, "Now they[3] have

---

3. At this point, the they in the dream became any or all people who wrongly thought they owned my (ie Teen's) house, the forces of shit out of luck mathematics, my own sensed but not articulated unworthiness, and/or all the things between me and being at the cottage. You know, "they."

to let me in." Ran upstairs to book the house. Clicked on the book-marked website. This:

SOLD--$630,000 10/27/17.

Panic. E-mail.

> To whom it may concern,
>
> I was in the process of booking this property for a rental early summer 2018, when I saw that it was sold. I am still very interested in booking the house, as my grandparents built it, and I have received a research grant to come, and work on a memoir about my time there. Could you please let me know if the new owner plans to rent, and if so put me in touch with them or whoever is handling that for them?

Then, snail mail:

> To the new owners of 209 Nubble Road
> From Kelley Jo Burke
> Re: Still a rental property?
>
> To the lucky new owners,   Dec 4, 2017
>
> Sorry to trouble you, I just wanted to enquire about your recent purchase of 209 Nubble Road. My grandparents built that house, and I'm a writer, and was recently funded to come down to Maine, and rent it as a part of my research for a memoir. After having the funding approved, I went back to complete the booking, and found it had been sold to you. Congratulations to you, and oh dear, a little, for me.
>
> I can make other plans for my research, but before I do, I thought I would check on whether you were planning to continue occasional rentals of the property.
>
> I have no wish to disturb you, and perhaps your plans are not yet set. But before I commit to a different place, I thought I would make sure that the house would not be available for rent for no less than 4 days and no more than a week after May 26 and before September 8. My research trip is currently scheduled for the last week in May, but I can certainly re-arrange travel plans. I can provide a cash down payment as soon as you need it, of course.
>
> This is certainly not your problem, but if you are planning to use the house as a rental at all, it would be a huge benefit to my research to be

able to stay in my childhood summer home.

Best, and happy holidays to you,

Kelley Jo Burke

(Ernestine and Jim Adams' grand-daughter)

Cold calls to the seller. Cold calls to the agency acting for the buyer. Silence. Weeks of. I cried. Booked at the hotel up the hill from the cottage. Wondered if I could even use the grant money that way. Whether I would be able to bear being up the hill, staring down at the cottage, where I could not go in.

And then in one day, this:

Hi Kelly Jo,

I am writing in regards to you staying at 209 Nubble while you gather info for the book you are writing. The owners would be delighted for you to stay at the property! I am not sure if my assistant... reached out to you already so my apologies if I am duplicating her work! What are the dates you would be staying?

Thanks,

Heidi (Williams Realty)

And this:

Hi Kelley Jo,

I'd like to introduce myself. I'm Gabrielle ... My husband and I purchased 209 Nubble Rd in York about 6 weeks ago.

I understand you are the granddaughter of the original owners and that you are going to be renting the house and writing a memoir.

If you didn't believe in God's goodness before ... I hope you will now.

I'm writing to let you know that when we went through the house we found some old things in the attic. Some had a lot of mold but some were in pretty good condition.

... I wondered if I could find a descendant of Jim Adams. (I didn't know your GM's name) I'm on ancestry.com and thought that might help me. At first attempt I could not find any info on a Jim Adams in York. I had decided to give the items to the York Historical Society if I continued to hit roadblocks.

I boxed up the items in the meantime, and at the time of your original inquiry I thought the items had been accidentally thrown out. I was heart-broken for you. I even went to the dump to see if I could retrieve them but was told that the trash had already been burned. I couldn't believe that after 60 years in the house, these treasures were accidentally discarded and then 2 weeks later we hear the granddaughter was coming and writing a memoir no less!

But that's not the end of the story ... (I'm giving you the blow-by-blow details since you are a writer, and I thought you'd like them).

Today I found out that my husband had moved the items to the old wooden chest we found! You have no idea how relieved I was!

So you see, God is good.

Merry Christmas,

Sincerely .... Gabrielle

Oh Gabrielle, you could not have written to anyone less convinced that God was good. Or there—at all. But today, you have made me see some kind of light.

Oh Gabrielle ... you're going to let me in.

What I Mean When I Say At The Lighthouse 2020[4]

So, to be clear, what I mean when I say "at the lighthouse," is "at my Adams grandparents' summer (ultimately year-round) cottage with this view of this lighthouse which is called the Nubble:"

---

4. ...was originally the title of this book. I thought it would work as a shout out to Virginia Woolf's much better book To the Lighthouse, and, you know, scent my pages with some literary knock-off perfume. Because let's be honest, this memoir needs some kind of hook. I'm white and mostly fortunate. As material for non-fiction—it's a nonstarter. But my publisher thought that rather than reference one of the most brilliant writers of the 20th century, something more representative of...well...me might serve better. Which is a little hurtful, but let's move on.

My parents moved from Adams Street when I was three. Again, from another place in Massachusetts to Canada when I was six. I moved again at seven, thirteen, fourteen, and then I started moving on my own at seventeen and so on, and so on. I have never received a satisfactory answer for the question, "Where's home?" except this view.

There's a theory that young children imprint on an environment the way they imprint on a mother's face. That there's a low frequency alarm that sounds at the back of the mind of those who are not where they initially registered as home. That's what I am experiencing when I am not at this place looking at this view. Hearing a tiny little voice screaming "NOT SAFE! WRONG! WRONG!" *all the time.* It is palpable. An ache. A gnaw. My little-bit-of-crazy, surging push to return to mothership.

I think it started here:

It is 1963 and I am less than two in this picture. It is the first concrete memory I have of being at the lighthouse, which means, in this case, on the rocks, below the cottage, which sits on a point a quarter mile to sea, and directly across a small straight *from* the lighthouse, seen in the view above. At the moment of the photograph's taking I already knew it was *my* rock. Just like the seagull behind, whose name was Oscar (he will be one of a thousand Oscars), was my gull. And the big ocean all around. All mine.

(The lighthouse was not mine. It was only itself's. And it looked after me, and that was as it should be.)

Oh look at you Kelley. Aren't you good? Aren't you smart? Teen pipes like a shore bird as this picture is taken. And I know that is true, and part of why all this is mine.

I can feel everything about this moment as I sit at my desk more than fifty-five years later. The rock's rough, sun-baked grate on my bare legs. The edges of those socks are gathered and the elastic leaves marks on my ankles over which I love running my finger. The white leather baby shoes make a satisfying, muffled thud when thumped together. The ruffled pleats on the front of that dress that are best seen, criss-crossed and ribbed, from inside the dress as it

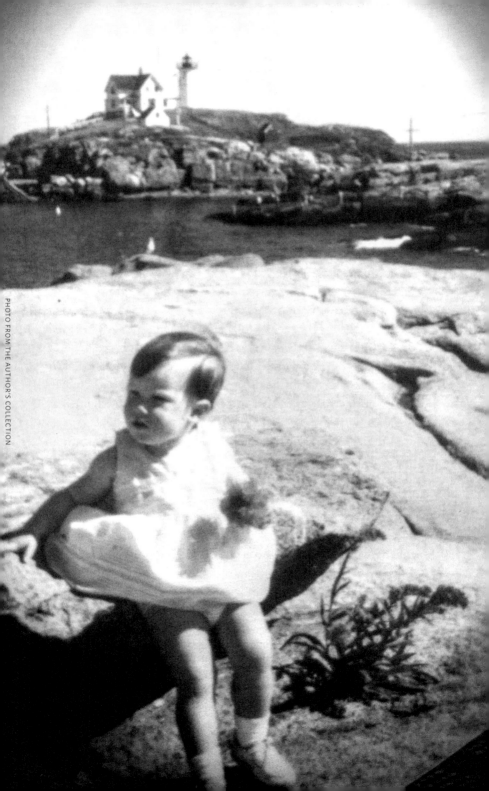

was pulled over my head, particularly when the sun shines through. I have ruffles on the diaper pants too ... and the sea breeze is lashing my hair into my already sun-squinted eyes. I belong in this place. It is glad to have me. I feel all that. Now.

What I can't feel is anxious. Because I'm not. There is no memory of being frightened in that moment. And I do not feel anxious now as I remember being there.

For the child in the picture, not being anxious is already the exception, not the rule. She will have her first, full-recall, crushing anxiety nightmare/panic attack less than a year after this is taken. It will involve a rushing tide that she viewed in a floor soap commercial. The soapy wave in the ad was exactly like the white booming breakers she watched from a distance at the beach. But the wave on the TV did not resolve into a harmless lace edge over toes. It surged through a house and over the kitchen floor, pulling back to reveal the lino gleaming.

"Waves can come into houses? Do we know about this?" my baby brain must have asked. In my resulting nightmare, the wave doubled down—thundering up the cellar stairs, flooding the kitchen, chasing me through the house, relentless and huge.

A grandfather clock—a singular six foot tall timepiece with an ornate and living face—waited at the end of the hall. I scrabbled hickey-dickory up, the waves hard behind me, looked to the clock face for help. But it scowled as I clung to its hour and minute-hand moustache. Looking down from what seemed a great height, I watched the white froth slap and suck below. It would sweep away all when it pulled back. And I could only hang on for so long.

I am going to feel like this most of my life: full of hanging on. Full of fear the way I am full of blood. At nine I will be so covered in cortisol-driven psoriasis that each night my hair will have to be soaked loose from my pus-covered neck. By twelve I will have my first dissociation episode, becoming catatonic with fear and just sort of checking out (my husband will later call it my "Kelley's drowning" face). By fifteen, I will be self-medicating. And by twenty-one, I will be a bulimic, promiscuous, knotted, inflamed sentient rash. Smells will explode my head. Sounds will make me faint. Regular pain will be intense pain, and intense pain will put me into shock.

(If I was ever to be tortured for information, I would confess. Immediately. Like right here. To you. Before I even started to *imagine* the pain. Before writing that sentence. Or this one. Before anything about anything brushed up against my broken glass and battery acid electric highway. Nope. Let's not go there. I'll confess. I did it. I know the codes. Hoffa's body is exactly where you think it is. I'm the Golden State Killer. I have Amelia Earhart's bones right here.)

Anxiety doesn't mean being worried. It means your body *knowing* that you, or someone you love, will die, in the next moment. Knowing that several times a week. Even as you also know that your body is a liar. Your blood sugar levels shoot up, pupils dilate. You sweat, heart pounds, mouth full of dust, and every muscle in your body seizes. And if you don't get a hold of it right away, you get some or all of: dizziness, hyperventilation, the conviction that you are choking on something, genuine chest pains with all the trimmings (aches in the arm, numb jaw, sometimes vomiting). I've fainted in an attack twice, both in very public places.

It will be *decades* before I understand that not everyone is like this. That most of you don't walk into a room and instantly run a mental movie of everything upon which you could impale yourself before reaching the couch. You don't say a silent goodbye to loved ones every time you go over a bridge, or, when there is an unexpected ring at the door, *automatically* picture a cop on the other side, the look on their face as they say that someone irreplaceable is now ground round on some highway, and can you identify the body? I didn't think so.[5]

But here, in this place, at this moment, at the Nubble, the anxiety that is already making me a nervous wreck ... stops.

---

5. I wasn't given medication for stopping panic until I was in my fifties. I took a tiny pill and then ... you get to feel this way all the time? You aren't scared except when there is something real to fear??? Why aren't you all just bursting into song? Randomly hugging each other? Making world peace?

My ruffled butt on this warm rock has decided that bad things can't happen here. I am full of sun and surf and relief, not in my heart—screw my heart—but deep, deep in my belly and groin, a huge released-by-terror pleasure that I will crave like a drug for the rest of my life.

Even looking at a photograph triggers that relief a little ... want to see another one?

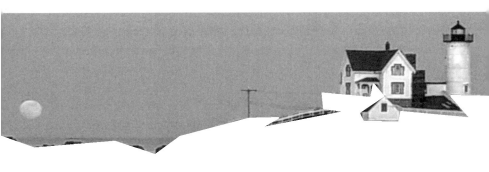

That's better. I can just keep them coming. I have a lot.

I have been told that the Nubble is the most photographed lighthouse in the world, though I am not sure how that would be measured. Certainly there are always people in Sohier Park, just off the Nubble, snapping pictures of the lighthouse as it sits on its cormorant- and-gull shit streaked rock pile, so close to the point that, at lowest tide, you can carefully walk from rock to barely submerged rock, to the island. It's not a great idea, and people drown in that little strait. But there was a famous keeper's cat that made the crossing regularly. And deer tap toe over too, tempted by the Nubble's quiet green spaces, only to regret it come high tide.

You *can* walk to the lighthouse. Only you *may* not ....

Only a chosen few, the keeper, and the maintenance crews, are ever allowed on Nubble Island. In the long past, there were keepers who augmented their Coast Guard incomes by conducting private tours. There's none of that now; it's a heritage site, and closed to the public. Every day, dozens, sometimes hundreds of pictures of the view of almost-to-the-lighthouse are taken and posted and shared, and these days, there are drone images, and video walk-throughs of the actual lighthouse home and tower posted by the keeper, all of which I stare at and replay, so much so that it seems I *must* have been there — at least once. I can tell you the slant of the grass. Where to place your feet on the wooden steps up to the lamp in the light tower. Come in. Let me make you a coffee. I know which cupboard it's in.

And yet not. So I cling, by way of pictures all over my house. Paintings. Charms. Coasters. Bookends. A pair of socks with the Nubble sprinkled over the cheap, stretchy made-in-china material, worn full of holes and darned with duct tape until I can wear them no more (I've started to react to the adhesive). I cling to this single memory of sun and rock and gull. Clutch to it like St. Ignatious' septum bone, a reliquary to miraculously slow my anxious breath.

So yes, obsessive. A little. A lot. You want to look at another one?

This is not from the porch, and was taken when I was not there.

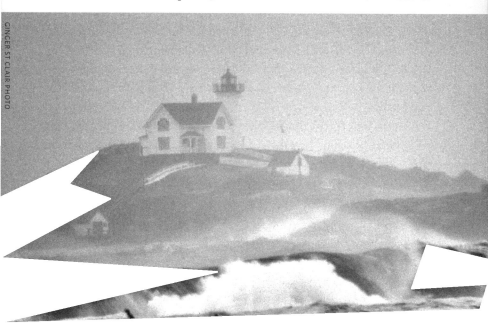

But I like this one because it's more like what the Nubble really is. It's not sunny that often. It's not collectible. Or cuddly. It is serious. It means business. It persists because it is a place where people who need to be saved, are.

For over a hundred years, it has kept ships from wrecking on Cape Neddick in the sticking-its-chin-into-any-coming-storm southern tip of the state of Maine. The keepers and their families were exceptional people, brave, cheerful, rash free, *good* people, who would slide a peapod boat, small, double-pointed, wooden thing like a dory, open and low-riding, down a ramp from the boat house, and launch into that, to try to save people.

In 1977, when NASA sent Voyager II into space to photograph the outer solar system, it was loaded with things designed to teach extraterrestrial civilizations about our planet. This included a picture of the Nubble. We wanted to teach E.T. that, among other things, we were keepers. People who give warning. Stand watch. Pull the wrecked back from the dark empty, and have hot rum and blankets waiting. (I mean, if you're trying to impress aliens, why not lead with your long suit?)

Babies were born in that house. People got married. Those who grew up a keeper's child describe their Nubble home as idyllic, paradisiacal—early rising to gull scream to see to the light and (in earlier days) the fog bell. Fishing. Duck hunting. Simple play in the salt air. Jolly times by lamplight. Riding flying boxes through the air to school. (I haven't shifted from the pastoral to Harry Potter—this is a true thing.)

Before we left for Canada, when I was five and still regularly going to my grandparents' cottage, a keepers' son named Ricky lived on the Nubble. There was and I think still is something on the Nubble, called "the bucket," a wooden box on cables used to shuttle supplies to the lighthouse from the mainland. Ricky's mom P. Jaye was not keen on using the peapod boat to get Ricky to school. The slide down from the boathouse could be unpredictable, the swell between the island and the rocks more so. And, depending on the tide, there was little in the way of safe landing on the other side. So she packed Ricky and a spare set of clothes, as the spray often completely soaked him before he made the other side, into the bucket. And cranked him across. Easy peasy.

Until someone realized that a kid in a bucket was quaint and news. And the papers, including the *Boston Globe*, got hold of it:

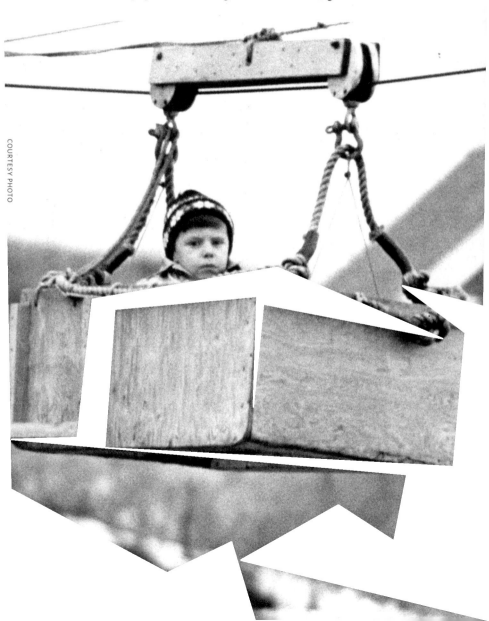

And then the jig was up. Someone at the Coast Guard saw how the sublimely unconcerned and life-jacket-free Ricky was getting to school every day. Stopped the whole thing. Ricky boarded in town during the school year. And being childfree became a job requirement for the next keepers.

When I was little, I wanted Ricky's life. I wanted to be the keeper's daughter. Because the keeper's daughter would feel like I did on the rock, *all the time*. Life on the Nubble would make her smart and pretty and serene and brave and game as a pebble, and so *not* what I was.

She would save people. Not constantly need to be saved.

I wanted that. I wanted it so badly that years later I erased Ricky when I told the story of the keeper's kid, made it a girl, sitting calm and slightly confused as to why anyone would think sitting in a bucket merited a picture, because after all how else was one to travel, except swaying in wave-roar air over black rock and kelp, bundled in boiled wool, hat firmly fixed against the nor-east wind that whipped over the hundred feet between the point and the island? Ricky had a younger sister, but it wasn't her I put in the box. My keeper's daughter was the eldest child in her family, equal parts Pippi Longstocking, Rapunzel, and Anne of Green Gables, and looked a bit like me.

When I would visit, during his time there, Teen kept saying she would have Ricky over to play with me. But in some sliding door way, it never happened and his family got kicked off the Nubble after the bucket solution was outed. So, despite the rom-com potential, a girl obsessed with a lighthouse, a boy in a box who I knew would understand that the girl was meant to ride the bucket with him, I never got to the Nubble by way of Ricky. Still I wish I had played with him once. It would have been like hanging with the Beatles.

Ultimately, I didn't want romance. I wanted how I felt when I was at the lighthouse. I wanted my pulse's anxiety-driven staccato to reset to the blink of the red light and the fog horn's steady purpose. I wanted the lighthouse to see me. And say, a la Peter Gabriel, "Grab your things. I've come to take you home."

You know, to the lighthouse? Where I've never been?

You see my dilemma?

The Chair 1996

When I get back from throwing the whales in the water and enter the cottage, the only thing that's changed is that the old man's reached over, turned out the light beside his chair, and settled in for the night. He thinks I've gone back to the hotel that he cries about every time he remembers that I've booked into it rather than stay with him. He's not hurt. Just angry at the waste. There are two unused bedrooms in the cottage. It's just stupid.[6]

I made placating noises about not wanting to put him to trouble. Fact is, the stench of the place is unbearable. As mentioned, the anxious tend to have an acute sense of smell. The better to sniff out fire, flood, poison, intruders, any of the fiercer animals, and past the expiration date food that will almost definitely kill us. Unfortunately is does not turn off. I often resort to what I call the Silence of the Lambs solution, which is to put Vicks VapoRub under my nose — I figure what's good enough for Clarice looking at a decayed body is good enough for me dealing with your poor cologne choices. On this trip, I'd left my Vicks at home.

---

6. Stupid is biggest word in the Adams world. It is the worst thing something can be. Worse than sinful. Worse than cruel. And there's a lot of it because so many people aren't Adams. Stupid is fools and chumps and Democrats and tourists. Oh, and because of her raging anxiety, Teen. Which makes the part where I am, in the family's estimation, "just like Teen" ... problematic.

The old man has some kind of hired help, but it seems not to be the kind up to cleaning a 900 sq. ft. bungalow. On Grampa's instructions, the cleaner has used only Liquid Gold on the furniture, panelling, and cupboards, as Teen did. But he doesn't remember, or never knew, that Teen also stripped the wood of its old Gold by scrubbing with Pine-Sol, before she re-coated it in the viscous mix of petroleum, mineral oil, and wax. That she spent hours over the maple tables and pine walls, keeping them gleaming and armoured against damp salt air. He simply tells the housekeeper to use the stuff, and she does, right over last week's coat. The result is a rancid punk of grease and dust on every inch of wood in the cottage. There is nowhere to rest a hand that does not leave a sticky brown mark on the palm, and a sticky, brown smell up the nose.

But that is not the worst of it. The La-z-Boy's the worst of it.

The one thing the housekeeper can't clean is the recliner, as the old man won't get out of it when she comes. The general musty-sweet smell coming from it, which one associates with the elderly, is wildly overwhelmed by a top note of urine. Lots of urine. Since Teen's death, I figure he's spent 90% of his time in the chair and not nearly enough showering. Or, I fear, toileting.

Confirmation comes as I stand in the dark looking at him. He wakes a little before he does it, stirs, shifts, and clearly considers whether to get up. Puts his spotted hand to the crank at the base of the chair. Takes the hand back, rests it on his chest, index finger tapping. Then a vengeful grunt, deep in the back of his throat, and the warm hiss. He doesn't know I'm watching. I think.

The chair, intensified by this most recent damping, is now a veritable censer of piss. I'm not going to sleep in this cottage. I don't want to eat here. I can barely breathe.

Opening the windows and airing the place is not an option. I'd tried earlier in the day.

"Teen-Ruth-Kelley leave that alone. I don't want 'em open." And Grampa stands, pulls the blinds down.

So I sit in the hot, dark, stinking house, straining to hear the sea, keeping my feet pressed to the floor so I can at least feel the rumble of the breakers through the boards. Remind myself that this is not a sight-seeing mission. This is a dealing-with-your-suicidal-grandfather mission.

He chose a good day, less than a year after Teen died, sunny with a breeze, high tourist season. He sat on the porch in the folding chair closest to the neighbours, and raised the gun to his head.

"It's no good, no more." Over and over.

The neighbours called the police. And the police called my mother in Winnipeg. And she called me. And I ferreted out the number of what's now called the Office of Aging & Disability Services in Maine. And state workers started to look in on him, though they kept the inadequate housekeeper. Despite her age and deficiencies, she was white. After listening to Mr. Adam's views on race relations, the service felt she was the best fit.

However, the resulting care did not include my mom, whose duty it was to come home and tend to him, give him some one to shout at, at the very least. So the gambit was not a success. He went back to crying and pissing in the blinkered and sealed cottage. Alone.

As the calls from the York Beach sheriff became more frequent, I started saying, "think I need to go down and check on him." Seeing normal people (like my husband) nod, yes, that's what you do if your grandfather is alone and in distress, made this seem more real, good and proper. Still, at the back of my head was a voice screaming as from a great distance that there was something here *not* good or proper. Not at all.

I was in my kitchen in Regina when I got the call from my mother about Teen. Late summer air heavy on my face, I listened to Mother's bald description of events: Teen had a habit of mixing up her pills, and then taking them all at once, and OD'd. Again. Needed flushing out at the hospital. This time, she got pneumonia as well. She was being treated for that, and then ... Grampa did what he did. And then, no doubt, went back to the chair to wait for the world to go back to what he required.

And all I could think at that time was, yup. Makes total sense. But there was a gumminess between my ears, leaving the question "what makes total sense?" to bounce at the entrance of my brain like a forgotten wind-up toy.

Almost a year later, I travelled to Maine to "help." And I double-hugged myself, because I was doing a normal thing and because I there was a good and legitimate reason to spend our nonexistent money to go to the Nubble.

Two days before, I'd arrived with a vision of my visiting self, a sweet-faced, caregiving grand-daughter, tripping through sunlit rooms, placing fresh flowers in whale-shaped vases, making wrongs right, like changing the linen or raising my grandmother from the dead.[7] A vision that quickly died in the breathless box in which I found myself.

Reminders of my (apparently actually dead) grandmother were *everywhere*. Her tall glasses in the cupboard, hand painted with Audubon birds, matched by swizzle sticks shaped like canes, tiny glass whistles dangling from each. The balls of Castile soap, untouched in their bowl in the bathroom. The pastel drawing of me as a child that she'd pointed at the last time I visited, saying, "That's my grand-daughter. She's a playwright." I allowed how I knew that, as I *was* her grand-daughter. She looked at me, taking that at face value since, with her brain in the state it was, she couldn't do much else. "You're a *writer*?" She widened her eyes, and put her hand to her chest. Gave me a little bow, as to a queen.

Teen's memorial consisted of a few people standing around in the cottage, over Grampa's objections. And the chair. I didn't have the thousand dollars to fly to Maine on short notice, and my folks couldn't afford to buy me a ticket. So I asked her minister to read this:

---

7. Assuming she was dead. That wind-up toy was still bashing on the limits of my understanding.

Letter to the guests (August, 1995)

As I am far away, I must thank you all for coming together to say good-bye to Teen in this way. I hope someone has said something about Teen's work for the communities she lived in and her joy in her friends and church. I don't know very much about that, because mine is a child's knowledge of Teen as we have lived apart for many years, and the visits were brief.

So it is of a child's understanding of her that I would like to speak. It is a privileged view, because as her grandchild, I think I got to see some of the best of her.

When I was very small, and was her neighbour, Teen would put my "little hand" in her "big hand" and walk me to the library. I cannot tell you what I had for breakfast two days ago, but I can tell you what each stone in the wall I walked atop on the way looked like, and I can feel the safety of being in that big hand, without any effort at all.

I can see every bit of the room you're standing in, though what I see bears little resemblance to its present incarnation. I can tell you exactly where the great conch shell used to sit on the shelf below the window, where the horseshoe crab hung in the net on the wall ...

I have only to close my eyes, and see Teen's strong arms throwing day-old bread to the gulls on the roof of the cottage, or digging with the poking stick as we walked Long Sands, giving me the words that have come to mean home: periwinkle, Mexican Hat, high tide, sandpiper, razorback, urchin, starfish, gull.

She gave me other things, an open and perhaps too easily moved heart, her dry wit, and the recipe for a superb highball. More than anything she gave me her unconditional regard — I have never been so smart or good-looking as when I was with my grandmother. I pass these things on to my children now, in full knowledge that I am merely delivering a gift from Maine.

I didn't go for her but I have come for him. Why? There's nothing here but the chair, the stink and the unprocessed thought that I am *late*, surging up from below, threatening to breach and set me a-founder.

I try to let charity reason with the scream that forms in my throat every time I crane my neck and fail to see the lighthouse through the draped windows. Old men dislike drafts. Bright light hurts their eyes. And I am supposed to be here for him.

Then I see him glance over his shoulder at the sea, screw up his mouth, look away. And I get it. He's not too frail for the light. Too chill for the breeze. He's jealous. And embarrassed. It's not that he doesn't want to look. It's that he does not want to be seen.

He loved who he was in this house. A born shop teacher, whose mother made him quit college and come home to respectable work as a banker and attention to her, he left his suits behind here. Been what he always wanted to be, a man good with his hands. Good at the potter's wheel, down cellar, the kiln's heat countered by the salt wind coming through the ground-level door. Good with repairs, at his huge, byzantine, every-nail-screw-and-tool possible, hooked or jarred, every blade honed to deadly edge, workbench. Good in a boat, pulling lobster and mackerel, watching green waves swallow the bow whole, doing no more than lash his young granddaughter to a railing and chuckle grimly with an eye to the shore. He loved his days here, being whole and useful and right.

It's not that Grampa'd gotten old. He was always old. He was old when he was young, a balding, moustachioed prince of New England at thirty, holding up his latest kill for the camera, replete in his sporting tweeds. Middle-aged before he was a third through his years. (Besides Adams men are absurdly long-lived. My great-grandfather Frank died up on his roof at 99-and-a-half years of age, replacing a shingle).

It's that he's not what he was. He can't go out on the boats anymore, his arthritis makes him too unsteady, and the friends who would take him out are dead. His wheel has stopped (he gave pottery up after producing yet another batch of brittle over-fired pots, too angry-impatient to kiln them low and slow—and now he hardly goes down cellar at all. Teen's loom is still there).

But the ocean is still what the old man was. Strong. Ungoverned. Indifferent to anything but its own will. The lighthouse, braced and taking all the sea can hammer, is more than he will ever be again. He doesn't want either of them. Gloating. Seeing him so reduced, so alone, sobbing on the porch, with a pistol that he can't seem to fire fallen to his soiled trousers. They can go to hell. The whole time I am here, I never see him open the blinds. He keeps the chair towards the TV and the volume good and loud.

Was the tide in when Teen died? I remember that was my only coherent thought, hanging up the phone, after Mom's call. I could bear it, I thought, looking out at the August heat ruin of my gardens, if, as she was dying, Teen could hear that she was where she loved the most. By the sea that she woke to each day like a young girl finding her beloved sleeping on the pillow beside her. Where her only charge was a gang of gulls who came to dinner daily up on the roof, gobbling the day-old Wonder Bread kept in a box just for them, webbed feet scrabbling, their cry, cackle, and murmur so reverberant that, when standing beside her, squinting against the brilliance of the sun-lit shingles they clattered on, I had a sense of the two of us held in a room made of gull voice.

I could bear it, if she knew she was at the Nubble.

But a day into this visit, it's clear to me that the old man went about then as he is now, closing windows and blinds as his wife rattled and stretched in her search for air.

And he's buried her in Westminster, away from the sea.

I understand that he is probably clinically depressed. I understand that fear is at the bottom of his anger. Fear of being less than. Of being thrown aside. Fear gnaws and drives him every bit as much as it did his high-strung wife, every bit as it does me — it's just with him, the reaction is to pass the bite on to someone weaker. I look at him sitting in the stinking chair entirely and essentially of his own making and think of a photo of him at maybe three? Long straight bangs hanging down over exactly the same worried, mistrustful, how-are-you-going-to-fuck-me-over eyes he peers through today. So much that he does he does as that child.

It's just, I want to be at the Nubble. I want to sit in the cottage and look across and feel my fear melt, thaw, and resolve itself into a dew. I want it so much that my fists clench and long to swing.

I understand him. Very well. It's just, it's no good. On that we can agree.

Eric ... and Counting 2017

The problem with the miraculous is you can't trust it. Having been given the thick envelope, the miracle of Gabrielle, the possibility of walking through the cottage in Maine without committing at least a misdemeanor, of going *to the Nubble*—well, bit much eh? Bit too perfect. Sort of things the angels are sure to take away.

Yes, I said angels. In my defense, it has been noted with some dismay that something like 75% of Americans believe that angels walk the earth. People who operate heavy machinery or perhaps even nuclear missile double ignition keys *believe* that heavenly, be-winged beings are hanging out on Earth, probably at Starbucks, because you know it's warm and they have free Wi-Fi, actively intervening in individual human affairs. And despite being an empiricist, atheist, show-me-science gal from way back—I am part of that statistic. With one difference. Unlike most of the besotted, Mommy-didn't-love-me-but-my-angel-does types, I don't think they're clutching to my shoulder, all cued up to hit the harp alarm when I wander into trouble. I think they are jealous, vindictive, *mean* angels who watch from a great distance and wait for me to slip up, like vultures with better hair. Show them what I cannot live without so they can take it.

They did it with the lighthouse.

And I see how the angels will do it this time. I have been given something I want desperately. That I chase in dreams. That is an ache in my gut and a moistening of my mouth every time I imagine it. And to grasp it, I will have to make a trip that I might have been able to handle on my own 10 years ago, but now? I've been gimpy, one way or another for most of my life. A curved spine and lousy feet set me up. Three babies knocked me down. I walk with difficulty, lose feeling in my hands regularly, and have yet to shake the delusion that I am very strong—because I was, once, on a Thursday when I was 17—and so I hurt myself constantly. And I have a setback—and by setback I mean a flying fall on glare ice and into dachshund shit, which would have been HILARIOUS in a YouTube video but not so much when face down in the teeny tiny dung—and so my mobility kind of sucks. Plus I'm night-blind, and there's the whole anxious about ... *everything* thing. I can't schlep a computer, rent a car, and drive up the Maine coast on my own. I have not thought this through and am not very bright and will have to give the money back. And the angels will laugh.

"I'll come." says Eric.

Can I ask this? Ask my husband to cart my anxious, off-kilter, and, it has to be said, more than occasionally damp self,[8] someone who is basically *the worst traveller in the world*, to New England? Thus making all this possible and sticking it to those fucking angels? Nah. That is one too many miracles. I'm going get smited, for sure.

I'm already well past due. I started the day that way, before the news about the rental, before getting the thick envelope. Because I started this day like the last 12,000 and so days, with Eric still in the bed beside me. As opposed to on the road to Cuba. With our savings, my good London Fog roller case, and the younger, thinner

8. Yes, I said it—damp. I am through menopause. I had BIG babies with a man more than a foot taller than me. One baby came out sideways. My pelvic floor looks like a San Francisco bridge post-quake. I am leaky, dodgy, and potentially something far worse—I'm not going say what, but let's assume that if Leaky and Dodgy were Dwarves #8 and #9, unnamed Dwarf #10 would always carry a change of undies and a packet of Handi Wipes.

woman with the gift of silence and mad Gumby-flexible bedroom skills that I can only aspire to, that the jealous angels have put in his path. They've been biding their time for thirty-five years plus. But I know they are going to make their move some time. My current theory is that they think making me sweat it out, morning after morning, is crueler than just taking him.

Stupid, stupid angels.

It's December of 1982. I'm in a kitchen that is improbably comfortable. As is the large post and beam house that holds it. The house sits halfway up the mountain in West Vancouver, one of the richest parts of a rich city. Blackberry brambles and grape vines wind over its mid-century lines; massive pine trees give shade. An ice cold stream tumbling through the backyard throws me every time I wake to its unspeakably pleasant sound.

Ridiculous. And yet here I am, 21 years old, with Eric, all 6 foot four of him, resting his hands on my shoulders. I have found his chest, and it is the only place I have ever been that is like the lighthouse. Eric's heartbeat is my surf, Eric's warm chest my rock. I pull the lapels of his blue velour bathrobe up to either side of my face and close out the not-Eric world. I have lost this feeling once. I know better now; I am never coming out.

We've been making love for, conservatively, three weeks. We break for the occasional plate of eggs and Eric's job. My school work is forgotten. We try to go to see friends but end up half dressed and suspiciously moist when left alone for any length of time. I still owe an apology to ... well ... everyone we saw during that period.

I am so grateful that this all happened before Instagram.

He goes to work, and I am very bad about letting him go. When he comes back I am barely dressed in a borrowed shirt and red long johns. They are easy to remove, in the doorway, often as not. It's been like this since three days after our first date.

Eight weeks before, I made an inauspicious landing in Vancouver. I left Winnipeg to do my last two semesters at UBC, because, I tell people, I wanted the experience of a bigger campus. Which is a lie. I went to Vancouver for love. True love. Endless holding, caring, saving, making-sense-of-it-all, and never losing, and never-being-frightened-again true love. The kind that never wavers. Love that will change me from lost to found. Love that will make me feel safe and whole, as I have not felt since I left the Nubble. Love that will fix me.

The man I left Winnipeg for wasn't Eric. I loved a lot of men before I loved Eric. Often for less than 24 hours. But what I lack in persistence I more than make up for in intensity.[9] The one that wasn't Eric, the one that leads me to pack my bags, transfer my credits, and work all summer to be able to afford (not really) a year in Vancouver, seemed perfect for the true love position. His politics were 44k left-wing. He worked on a fishing boat (on the wrong ocean, but an ocean still). And he made love like a sea otter, happily rolling in the sunny brine of our sex.

We met at a conference. I stayed on longer than planned. We listened to Joan Armatrading, drank wine, and floated.

We agreed that we weren't into monogamy, that sex was friendly exercise, and wasn't it great not to be hung up. Then I moved to Vancouver to lock that sucker down.[10]

When I arrived the sea otter had someone else in his kelp bed.[11] I found this out by walking in on them.[12] Not, I suspect, because I surprised him but because he thought it best I find them like that.[13]

A few moments later, I sat in the house breakfast nook with one of the sea otter's housemates. The last time I sat here, I was

---

9. My counsellor says I use orgasms like vitamins—one-a-day to keep the banshees at bay. My old boyfriend gives a British-flavoured shudder and says that most round-heeled women stop to change the sheets occasionally. My flaky friend just shrugs and says, "Scorpio."
10. You can hear the angels rubbing their wings tips, sharpening them to razor points.
11. Whoosh—the angels pouncing—wing jab to the jugular.
12. Plop. Blood from my emotional artery spatters to the floor.
13. Flap. Huge black wings spread and lift off in victory.

eating pancakes wearing my beloved's fishing sweater, a pet girl in a houseful of guys. On this day, I talk through my situation with the housemate in a manner that I think is tough and unsentimental and must have been tragic and hilarious. I try to ask him to let me stay in the house, not with the sea otter, without asking him to let me stay. He listens with the same look he gives the marks at the carnival where he works summers, not unkind, just trying to figure out how anyone got this dumb, and says quietly, "There's a board with rooms to rent posted at the student union building." And then he leaves.

Staggering on my way out, bags in hand, I had to go back into the bedroom. Sea Otter asked me to drop his clothes at the laundromat. My father's voice, two years earlier while I still lived at home in Winnipeg, plays over and over in my mind as I look at the laundry bag.

I'd been stranded, miles and miles from our house. Two in the morning, missed the last bus, no change for a pay phone and by no means convinced my parents would come and get me if I did call. I'd flagged down a passing station wagon. A guy rolled down his window, not the late shift dad I hoped was stopping, but to all appearances sober, clean. Smiling. I told him the fix I was in, a little tearily. He said he would get me home. Turned up the heat in the car. Smiled again. And promptly tried to kidnap and rape me.

After the whole, "let me out, let me out here, please let me out or I will jump out" conversation, I walked the rest of the way home, cold, weeping, shoes wildly inadequate. Until I finally stood sobbing in the parents' bedroom doorway, gasping out what almost happened.

"Serves you right. Maybe next time maybe you'll know better," said Dad, rolled over and fell back asleep. Some pushed-back-in-the-corner part of me whimpered. The rest of me agreed.

Holding the sea otter's laundry, I think: serves me right.

So? I was twenty. I made a fool of myself over a boy. I lived poor and believed I had no friends, along with almost everyone who leaves home young without enough money. Whatever. I was neither beaten nor homeless nor downtrodden in any real way. I was simply, profoundly lost and disgusted with my own inability to rise above being lost. Is it any wonder that I have a hard time believing that what happened next was anything but a mistake?

It is two weeks into the disastrous move to Vancouver, and I sit in the student newspaper office, trying to stiff upper lip my way through the semester. Someone stands in front of the copy edit desk. I recognize this with a repressive "Hey. What can I do for you?" and continue, head down, vindictively red-penning.

"Um," he sounds more surprised than pissed off, but I lift my head, smelling an error in process. Look. Holy shit. A towering ginger in a sky blue ski jacket. Rugby shirt and pants. I've grown up with dogs. I am shit with people, but dogs I know. And this, my friends, is a good dog. Kind. Decent. Ironically wistful. Second (and third and fourth) thought careful. And smart.

Lower my eyes again, quickly. No way. I am no longer looking for love. Or heart's-ease. Sweaty, high-IQ virgins who can tell you who played bass on the 1973 Lou Reed in Amsterdam bootleg version of "Sweet Jane" but not what one does with a clitoris are my wheelhouse, and serves me right — for wandering afield of that.

"I'm visiting. I'm ... I was the photo editor," he says, smiling. Right at me.

There is a change in the no-longer-looking-for-love plan.

"Who's that," I ask my friend Muriel as he goes to talk to the rest of the staff, all of whom know him better than they do me.

"Eric Eggertson," she says.

"I'm going to *get* him."

She stares. "I think he's living with someone."

"What's your point?"

Turned out his girlfriend recently left him for the architecture department. I didn't know that. I didn't care. I put my one and only go-to plan into action, the one I have because I'm smart and chubby and angels hate me so I have to come with value-added: I ask him out and make sure that he has *absolutely no question* that there will be sex at the end of the night.

We arrange a midnight breakfast date on my birthday, as I will be working that night at College Printers, where the UBC student newspaper is produced. The 'round the night shift paste-up was routine for Eric; after leaving UBC for a real job at a real newspaper, he would still sometimes drop by with cappuccinos from Joe's (the best coffee in Vancouver) for the production crew.

He shows. Hands me a coffee. Stands beside me as I proof the waxed pages of copy that we will roll on newssheet-sized manila boards and send to be converted into actual newsprint. I show off my butch, ink-smeared skills while trying to be clear about the whole absolutely-no-question thing. You know, accidental lean-ins. Eye contact. Lip licking. I may have even passed him a note.

Nothing. No reaction at all. He leaning over the pages I'm proofing, pointing to something I've missed. What the hell? I hum as I work harder—"You Can't Hurry Love"—trying to steady my nerves. But I know to the bottom sticky dregs of my gut that I am mistaken. My sexual availability is not sufficient recompense for my basic loser-dom. Again. My heart starts to pound, and the shame I felt when I walked in on Sea Otter and friend rises burning in my throat. I bend over the sheet of paper and hide a sob.

"I was alone, I took a ride, I didn't know what I would find there," I hear him singing Beatles under his breath. "Got to get you into my life." Oh. The blood leaves my plummeting gut, floods my face. I can hear the brass blast that should follow his sotto voce singing. It sounds like hope.

And then it's midnight, and all the printers' watches go off and they sing happy birthday to Muriel and I (we share a birthday, they are actually singing to Muriel, who everyone knows, and I am getting the fumes, but that's okay with me). With a confirming look to Eric, and a self-conscious good bye to everyone (look the loser has a date!), I grab my coat, and we make to leave, heading for a quick breakfast and, as I am now daring to hope is understood on all sides, sex in the back of his car.

It is at this point that the Sea Otter[14] redeems himself. He'd been working on the paper that night as well, and, on hearing that Eric and I are going for breakfast, says something like "Great!" and grabs his coat. I look at Eric, and he at me, and there is a shared "Can you believe this?" that is instant, unquestioned, and direct; we have now known each other forever. We have a mind-reading level of intimacy.

I don't think s.o. was in any way suffering dumper's remorse. I think he was hungry.

So we *all* go for breakfast. And when s.o. is in the bathroom, Eric, who knows about s.o. and I — it's a newsgathering organization, everyone knows — without saying anything, reaches over and takes s.o.'s jacket. Stuffs it inside his own. Looks at me. And waits.

s.o. does not notice. Not when he comes back to the table. Not when we head out into the damp November night. Not when he climbs into the back of Eric's cold Volkswagen Beetle and waits to be taken home. I look at Eric and start to sing "my coat lies over the ocean, my coat lies over the sea …." Eric joins in, "oh bring back my coat to me." Nada.

We drop s.o. off. He climbs out the back. Shivers in what is now an icy downpour, and invites us in. We stay warm in the little car, staring at s.o., whose hair is flattening and shirt growing transparent in the deluge. Eric looks at me; I shrug. Eric reaches under his coat, pulls out S.O.'s jacket, gets out, and puts the coat over the soaked s.o.'s shoulders. Tears back to the car. Drives to my place. And we sit in the bubble of quiet held by the battering rain.

When we finally go in, I make him pot after pot of espresso, because it's all I have. And we talk. About all of it. About s.o. About the shame that was the first thing I woke to and the last thing I saw at night. About how I was pretty sure I should go back to Winnipeg.

He's kind and quiet and listens intently. And each and every

---

14. This is getting tiring. I'm going to abbreviate him: S.O.

moment that we talk, I wait. I wait for us to head downstairs to my cattle-pen single room in the basement that I rent from a bunch of yuppies' trying to cover their even-in-1982 impossible Vancouver mortgage and get on to the guaranteed sex.

At four in the morning Eric says, "I guess I better go." And the world that was slowly rebuilding around me clatters. What happened to "no question"? Crystal clear? I'm a sure thing. Sure things don't get passed over at four in the morning unless the guy finds you *repulsive*. I've been without enough money for food for months — I'm comparatively thin. Cheek-boney. I think the anemia makes me look soulful. What's wrong?

I stagger to the door, following his long, strong back. He turns in the doorway. "I'm glad you didn't go back to Winnipeg," he says. And he holds my gaze.

It can only be the flood of relief that allows me what comes next.

I lean against the door frame, take a beat long enough for a Lauren Bacall drag on a mental cigarette (I can't afford non-mental ones at this point). Say:

"I thought something would turn up."

Three weeks later I'm here, living in his house. I'm living in his blue velour robe and red chest hair triangle (he was more than a foot taller than me, and so my face to his sternum is ground zero when we stand together). The house, which he is minding for his father, is too grand to feel like anything other than borrowed, but this warm, dark compressed space, filled with the smell of him, fortress-like with his size and stillness, is mine.

I've got *it*. True love. Endless, holding, caring, saving, making-sense-of-it-all, never-losing, and never-being-frightened-again true love. The kind that neither wavers nor has to be won again and again. And I have done nothing to deserve it. There is nothing in my story to this date, there will continue to be nothing, which requires *this* ending.

I know dogs. And I know stories. Once upon a time there was a serves-her-right, high-strung, angel-harried girl who thought finding true love would *fix* her. That girl doesn't get the good dog, let alone the good man. She gets a sharp kick in the ovaries, and learns that she has to fix herself before she can even imagine a story with that ending. Right and proper. Women's Studies 101.

Clearly, I've got someone else's ending. Someone who ought to have this. Someone who ought to have him and is wondering what the hell happened. I almost feel sorry for her.

Almost.

Thirty-five years, six months, and twenty-two days later now and counting — and I do count. Every time Eric makes an offer like "I'll come," an offer that the person who is supposed to have him might deserve, but I certainly do not, I run the numbers. Wonder if this is the one that will push the angels into making their move.

It's only a matter of time, you see. I knew that thirty seconds after that moment in the kitchen, thirty seconds after the "I got it!" exultation registered and the fear flooded back in. I would lose this again. Because as much as I love him (and my god I do), and as much as he loves me (and by god, he seems to), I am not fixed. I am broken and at some point that will outweigh the love. And every time I ask more of him than I should, I push us a little closer to that inevitability.

I *know* that going to the Nubble for a week on a writing retreat isn't going be The Fix. But I believe that there is something that will happen if I can go in, be there, feel what that place makes me feel, stop hearing that "NOT SAFE! WRONG! WRONG!" alarm, which will show the way to being fixed. Safe. Angel-proof.

"I'll come," says Eric.

"Could you? Please?"

Four Other Things I Mean When I Say At The Lighthouse

"The lighthouse was then a silvery, misty-looking tower with a yellow eye that opened suddenly and softly in the evening.
... He could see the white-washed rocks; the tower, stark and straight;
... he could see windows in it ... so that was the lighthouse, was it?
No ... nothing was simply one thing."

To the Lighthouse, *Virginia Woolf*[15]

1. In the cottage.

I don't know how many times I have been at the cottage. The only time I visited regularly was between babyhood and the age of five, when I lived on Adams Street, and then later in Amherst, Mass. I believe we visited the cottage often during that time. But I may be wildly over-estimating the number of visits.

After the move to Canada, we, being my parents and my brother and the sister who joined the family our first year in Winnipeg, visited the cottage twice. And I was sent there on my own when I was

---

15. There. Snuck a little bit of Woolf in after all. I can feel the literary stock of this book rising.

eleven, because it seemed the only way get me to shut up about going "home."

After that there were six visits when I was an adult—two when I was single, two with my kids and Eric, two when I was dealing with the deaths in '96 and '97, and one where I just wandered outside the locked building well after it belonged to someone else, peeping in the windows and scared of getting shot—it is perfectly legal to shoot someone trespassing in the state of Maine. Doubly so if the trespass includes touching someone's lobster trap. And then, the writing retreat visit in 2018.

Despite having no idea how often I was there, the cottage is my memory palace. I can walk every step of its original incarnation, prior to it being winterized in 1972. That early cottage is made of wood and lino, and meant for summer. Fishing tackle behind the door, a net full of beach finds on the wall, more on the window ledges, a tin shower for rinsing sand from cracks and crannies. There's a square shelf nailed to the porch railing to offer gulls scraps, guts and the boiled-out contents of gathered shells. There is the smell of Bain de Soleil, and drying starfish. Squeal of lobsters contracting (not screaming) in the pot. Gush from the hose as sand is washed from small feet. And there is the Nubble blinking through the kitchen window as we played endless hands of late night crib.

When I *ache* for where I come from, I don't ache for where I was born or where family still lives. I ache for the cottage that the lighthouse watched over like an architectural rather than personified god.

So that's also what I mean.

2. On the rocks.

Edging the sea below the cottage is a line of massive rocks. The whole of Cape Neddick, where the cottage sits, is rocks, with the barest covering of thin soil, wild roses and morning glories. Where the soil peters out, and before the sea begins, the huge and weathered stones, beaten by fierce North Atlantic waves into old grey monster heads, too ancient to bother with anything as vulnerable as ears or eyes or nose, sit, taking in the sun and waiting for the next onslaught of water.

I learned how to climb those rocks early. I can't remember a time when I didn't know how to look for where to put a foot, where to brace a back, how to tell the safe from the slick. I know where you have to get past before tide comes in and between which rocks will be the miniature seas, made of a bit of weed, a few snails, some darting minnows, one starfish, held in a stony crevice and sufficient to themselves.

I do not know when I learned that. Or who taught me. I have just always known.

I am eighteen. Sun-burned and shagged-out, at the end of a summer job in Montreal, I have come down to Maine. Teen does not know how to have an adult version of me around. She will not let me walk Nubble Road without holding her hand. She would prefer me not out of the house at all. There is no end to it. "Oh honey, don't touch that. Oh Kelley, don't go over there. It makes me cry. It makes me cry to think of it. Watch when you cross. Stay out of the run-off water, it's dirty. Not the attic, honey — it is not safe. Let's get you in a shower. Do you need this? Put on a coat. Put on a hat. Careful on those stairs. I broke my hips on the rocks. Twice honey. Twice."

It's not my fault you go down to the rocks half-corked, I think. You're always half-corked. Yesterday, you drank me under the fucking table before *noon*. With the before lunch drink. The during lunch drink. The after lunch drink to hold us over until cocktails at four ... it was a hundred degrees, and I was blasted. I passed out by 2:30 and never got to my rock.

Anyway it is not going well. I call my mother to tell her my visit "home" is not at all what I expected. That Teen's crazy is in fact driving me crazy.

"Now you know what it's like," she says.

But I need to get to the rocks. I need to know if who I was when I was down on the rocks is still there. I wait until Teen is out getting the mail — no house delivery yet in York Beach, Maine, just an eagle embossed brass post office box with a satisfyingly heavy combination lock. Pull on my cool Quebecois flax pants and a plaid shirt stolen from one of the guys I'd been sleeping with, look Grampa in the eye and say, "I'm goin' down to the water."

He shrugs. The day before, when I headed to the rocks too drunk to climb but still aching to get close, I'd stood on the first flat boulder closest to the cottage, my rock in fact, spread my arms like the cormorants on the Nubble's point across from me, and, a little unsteadily, rejoiced. Then I'd heard the crack of a rifle. Sounds echo clearly off rocks. I turned to see him, peering, hunched like a vulture, bald head and all, aiming his double-barrel shotgun, the one loaded with buckshot and salt.

"Grampa it's me!" I'd screamed. He paused. Peered again.

"Kelley? That you?"

"Yes!"

"Put away the gun then."

He doesn't want to talk about the rocks.

I go down the path he made through the roses and poison ivy. Start to climb along the water.

Understand, everywhere else in the world, I am clumsy. Pathetically so. They called me Fairy Foot as a child, based on my staggering thunder up and down stairs. I will of course turn out to have been partially crippled my whole life, a shin-splinting, back curving, hook-footed mess, but as a child it is put down to my fat and my just-too-muchness and my utter lack of ladylike anything.

But this is me moving with ease and agility north around Cape Neddick and (I felt at the time) halfway to Ogunquit. There are scrapes and a tear in the knee of my pants and I do not care. Every move I know how to make tells me that I am where I belong. That this is still mine.

Which is when I find the guys. Four of them. European bathing suits, minuscule shiny triangles of cloth, over *impressive* packages. Bronzed skin, tight bodies. Two pretty. Two older, wearing heavy gold chains at neck and wrist. As a group they register the unkempt and hopelessly dowdy thing crawling towards them. Pretty One the First raises a perfect taffy brown arm and calls out, "Bloodies!"

And then I am sitting with these lovelies, chatting away, turning the past days with the grandparents into funny songs I sing for my Bloody Mary.

A boat sound. Not the chug and diesel of a make-or-break lobster boat, or the crisp clip of a pleasure cruiser. Something huge. White. Powerful. It's the Coast Guard. Cutting engines.

At this point, it bears knowing that for most of his time at the Nubble, my grandfather lived by the scanner. He listened to police, fire and the Coast Guard —confirming what he heard going on by regular peering through his magnificent telescope. He made regular contributions, reporting scuba divers troubling the traps studding the water between us and the Nubble. Bad drivers. People of colour — I will not use his name for them — but any people of colour. They had no business in York. Or Maine. Possibly the entire Eastern Seaboard. Maybe South Boston, so there could be maids and bus drivers, but if they showed up on Nubble Road, they were reported to the police. And the fire department. And the Coast Guard. He was asked to stay off emergency channels, but coloured people were an emergency, so what was their point?

Let's go back to the cutter. It hangs off the rocks. Someone on deck has binoculars. The lovelies, memories of bath house raids fresh, grab towels and blankets to cover their near-nude lolling selves. Binoculars grabs a megaphone.

"Kelley Burke?"

"Yes? " I shout.

"Your grandmother wants you home. You're late for lunch."

The lovelies' screams of laughter bounced off the stones, cast a thousand gulls into shade.

I grin. Start my climb back along the rocks, where my feet know what to do. Where I still belong.

So that's also what I mean.

3. With Teen

Barefoot and head down
beating the summer people to the tide's retreat
search for the sand dollar
with its story yet unbroken

Or crouching in a salt marsh
Birding sheet in hand
   Kelley look:
   A bittern
   a willet
   Oh
   those Blue-winged Teals

Or best
driving past the lighthouse
legs nicely toasted on the Saab's red seats
Teen shifts to neutral
and we glide
   uuuup
      and dowwwwn
the roller road
Can we make it to the driveway without gearing in?
Old woman and child
   frightened of every
      single
         thing
   careening cliffside
Wheeeeeeeee!

4. If It Stopped

I am itchy. And scratchy. And off.

Show me contentment ... and I'll poke it over. Point at the nasty that waits underneath. Gifts are for losing. Love's a landmine step. And serves you right, girl who is neither smart nor pretty, when it all goes/blows.

Then it stops. Just for a moment. Just enough to break my heart. And I think it will never be more than a moment, unless *I* stop. Altogether.

Then I think that it's best I don't think that way. So I think of something else.

I think of the lighthouse.

So that's another thing I mean.

Geld 1969

My dad stood staring at me, a mittfull of letters in his hand. I was kneeling on the closet floor, eyes squeezed shut, muttering the 23rd Psalm, which was the only God thing I knew. I kept my hands as close as possible to the position learned from the plastic replica of Durer's "Praying Hands" that my Burke grandparents gave me (they knew I wasn't baptized and so was probably going to hell, but that wasn't going to stop them trying). I looked up to see his face twisted in a familiar mix of exasperation, affection and guilt—guilt because he wanted to laugh, and laughing at a kid at prayer was definitely not best practice for an educational psychologist. Affection because he did like me. And exasperation because I don't think he believed for a minute that what he was looking at was an innocent child's turn to her Lord. It was guerrilla protest theatre, one tent in a whole carnival of crazy that I endured since our move to Canada, eight months before.

I have a vague memory of my mother and father telling me that we would be leaving Massachusetts and moving to Winnipeg. My professor dad needed a job with the possibility of tenure. In 1967, Boomer babies were flooding dug-out-of-the-mud Western Canadian universities and they were desperate for faculty, offering tenure for three unblemished years and ten Wheaties box tops. My mis-matched parents needed neutral ground on which to build their own family. Like other young liberals of the time, they decided to adopt a child of colour (ultimately my sister Jess), and that would go better away from the varying degrees of racist relatives. And then there was Vietnam and the draft, and lord knows how long that would drag on, and they had a son (brother Steve). So they decided on Canada the way you decide on boysenberry ice cream; you've never tasted a boysenberry, wouldn't know one if it bit you, but word is, it's nice.

Moving to a foreign land sounded very cool and storybook to six-year-old me. I imagined palm trees. I imagined monkeys. I quite fancied having a monkey. My cousins had one. There was a theme park in Vermont called Santa's Land, and part of that meant they had a chimpanzee named Sam who lived in the house, used the bathroom, and ate at the table. So this hope was more reasonable than it seemed, if geographically misguided.

It all seemed very exciting until the North American Van Lines semi dumped our stuff into a Winnipeg made of darkness and cold. And then something I had not considered came to me: I wouldn't be going to the Nubble that weekend. But surely, the weekend after?

Well no.

And so it began.

"I want Teen."

"Stop it Kelley."

"Take me home."

"You are home, Kelley."

"When are we going to the big ocean?"

"It is a very long trip. It will be a long time."

For a kid used to Massachusetts' comparative mildness, that first winter in Winnipeg was impossible. Implacable. They had to be kidding. Sent out to play in the snow, I was returned to my mother, teeth chattering, by our neighbor. "Why is she out in her fall coat?" the neighbor asked, staring at my only winter jacket.

Steve and I were hauled to the Army & Navy surplus store and zipped into snowmobile suits and boots which were stiff and ugly but, at a reasonable price, would keep us from dying. A furry blue knit scarf, wide enough to cover my entire face, double-looped above and below the eyes, completed my winter toilette. At -20 or worse (and it was always worse, winter of '67/'68, -50 for weeks on end, birds clattering to bits as they froze and fell mid-flap), it would be spangled with snot-and-breath-cicles, and painfully freeze to my lymph-weeping, raw upper lip.

I got sick. Constantly. Strep, Hong Kong flu, whooping cough, and something rheumatic that left me without the use of my legs for several weeks. It seemed the viruses of Canada saw my landed immigrant papers, screamed "we've got a live one!" and climbed into my orifices en masse. It must have been awful for my already gob-smacked mother, who surely was having her own what-the-hell-are-we-doing-here moments. Night after night of no sleep with a (maliciously?) sick kid, who had a habit of staring up through the fever sweat, eyes glittering and asking, "now are you going to take me home?" can't have helped. Meanwhile, my dad, fell victim to various 1970's pop psychologies, was trying to figure out how a now 7 year-old was manipulating her own immune system to such catastrophic effect.

I tried. I went to school and made it clear I was far too smart for the class I'd been put in via pointed and hammy yawns. Built on that killer plan for instant popularity by using my advanced vocabulary on the children of slaughterhouse workers and travelling salesmen. All things considered, took very few of the playground beatings I so richly deserved, and somehow made friends of sorts with Norma Kerr next door who was clever in a sweater-wearing and perpetually allergic way.

But then the inescapability of my situation would make itself felt and I was back to being that other kid, lonely, desperate, hard -done-by, and in constant protest. Freedom fighter, spiritual hermit, one-child band ... it was all pretty much the same impulse and it was constant. There was a hole in me that was plugged every time I was at the lighthouse, that was now wide open, and all the gnawing anxious animals were scrabbling out and over my skin, leaving it raw and weeping.

So yes. I was a flat out pain in the ass for two young parents who were also far from home, broke, and trying to process for themselves what they'd done.

I can't remember the details of the particular fight. I do know how it felt, because fights with Mom had a consistent, chewy centre for as long as we lived together:

ME: *I know what is best for me, and what is best for me is to go* **home**. *I am prepared to argue for it endlessly with my amazing, precocious, and inexhaustible words.*

MOM: *I am the mother. You are a child. You are done with that place and those people.*

ME: *Can't be. Won't be. Why and why and why?*

MOM: *Because I said so.*

ME: *I will now go to my well of inappropriately gut-wrenched emotion, and cry until I vomit. I am a free human being with an independent will, which I now exert.*[16]

MOM: (to my dad, with her eyes) *"Are you sure I can't hit her?"*

Dad generally started as Solomon, and finished as Samson, roaring and pulling down the temple. This time, after I was shouted and

---

16. There is a price to be paid for letting your child read Jane Eyre at 6 years old. Sure, great to bring up at parties, but you're going to get some epic literary rhetorical shit thrown at you.

banged into my room, the straw that broke the camel's-back-ishness of the situation came into focus. Reason and the inalienability of human rights would not move my oppressors. I could stay and live under tyranny or take arms against it, and strike out on my own. For someone who could at least argue for membership in the Daughters of the American Revolution—there could be only one course.

I pulled the North American Van Lines carton (taller than me) out from the corner and pushed in a few clothes and all of my stuffed toys. I dragged the box behind me, down to the front hall, and climbed into my snowmobile suit and boots. But before heading out, I thought of provisions, and headed for the kitchen.

"The food in this house is for people who live here," my father called from the next room. He was using his white lab coat voice, a let's-see-what-she-does-if-we-change-the-walls-of-the-maze experimental curiosity. I slammed the fridge, the first stab of worry replacing rage in my stomach. But I was committed, and pulling on my mitts, pulled the box out of the house and down the broken concrete steps into a black January night of killing cold.

The streetlights gave our warm-windowed, house-lined road the feel of being a hallway in yet another larger, colder house. With some basic notion of settlement being best made by water, I walked towards my schoolyard rink, box sledding behind me. I believe I thought I would cut ice and build an igloo by one of the nets.

Arriving at the rink, I registered the following facts: I had nothing with which to cut ice; I had no real understanding of how igloos were constructed; and fingers and toes could hurt in ways that I had not yet imagined. I fished around in the box for my pink flannel pajamas, sat down on the ice on the lee side of the carton, and wrapped my hands and feet.

And for a moment, it was … good. It was quiet. My house was never quiet, and the racket left me with a headache so constant I didn't register it as a condition. There was no one to look after, or resist. It was a house of ice and one cardboard wall, but it was mine.

Almost like my rock. My seagull. My ocean. I wondered how long I could stay there. What the kids from school would say when they found me living rough at the rink. I wondered, looking down Howden Road, the slow cold settling under the brilliant rink lights, when someone would come and get me.

It came to me then, massive and slow, like an iceberg pressing past the lamplights. No one would.

I would have to leave the rink — I could see that. I wasn't upset or embarrassed. Even with my ingenious pajama wrap, I didn't think I could make it through the night. I needed shelter and there was only one door that would open to me.

Norma Kerr's dad didn't even let me in. Norma was already in bed, and I wasn't getting her up. He put on his coat, grabbed the moving box and hauled me and it over to the concrete steps next to his. Grimly rang our bell.

My mother did not rise. I don't remember her speaking either, though it is possible that she was arguing, in whispers, for the Kerrs keeping me.

Dad took the situation in hand. Making eye contact with Mr. Kerr, he only half-opened the door and said, "People who live here can come in." I could see the clipboard materialize in his hand, as he prepared to record the results.

"I live here," I said. I was no hero. I didn't want to die. And the Kerrs clearly weren't in the market for a free-spirited foster daughter. I dragged my box to my room, eyes away from where my mother sat, and got a bowl of Rice Krispies.

What was left for me but prayer?

I had read *Little Women*, and was much taken with the section in which Amy is encouraged to set up a chapel in her closet as a source of calm and solace while away from her family. My single source of calm and solace was now 1,800 miles away, and it looked like it might take a little more time to get back there — so I needed a stand in. And I have to admit, Amy's chapel accessories attracted me:

a kick-ass gold and ebony bead rosary, dainty flowers, a painting of the Virgin Mary ... it sounded so classy, and like what a deep soul like me would have. (I was sure even in grade two that I was a deep soul, the girl who ordered not burgers but *Filet-O-Fish* at McDonald's, because she was a rebel, a dreamy eyed, book-loving, meant-for-something-special free spirit. And besides, fish came from the ocean and the ocean was where that girl should be. I also drank Dr Pepper. 'Nuff said.)

I didn't know that flowers could grow in Canada at this point. All I'd seen was a lot of bleak and frigid. So that was out. Also, rosaries were in short supply. Dad gave up Catholicism for humanist psychology and general grooviness and Mom was so very WASP. So fixing up my chapel was a problem. But then I saw an oddly groomed and emphatic man on TV offering a free plate depicting the rolling away of the stone after the Resurrection with the angel saying she was sorry but Jesus stepped out, could they call again? Just the thing to fill my chapel gap.

I mailed a letter to something called Oral Roberts University, and requested the plate. It arrived, mono mud-colored and heavy, made from cheap clay, but satisfyingly devout. It became the centre of my closet chapel, along with my Small Child's Bible—a beautiful blue hardcover edition that was my mom's, with the best illustrations of white people dressed like Middle Eastern people you've ever seen, wrestling lions and walking out of fire and hitting on doe-like women at oases wells. Also a quickly confiscated candle array—my family had no sense of ritual. Anyway, it was all behind the folding closet door, a little altar that I would sit in front of and pray for all I was worth. And then wait to be caught by the great hand of love.

Instead, I was caught by the hand of Oral Roberts. The letters my dad held were requests for "seed" from that august institution. Seed being cash. And while Luke 6:38 said, "Give, and it shall be given unto you," in the case of my plate, it had already been given unto me, and so it was time that I give something unto Oral. So he could continue to sow the faith in the (holy) state to which he was accustomed.

Life Lesson: There are no free plates.

This was nine months into the Canada experiment. Dad's guilt load was already at critical. He abandoned everything to make this leap into a different life. That he in some way broke, or at least bent, his first born child was not something I think he could take on at this or any moment. I could see him picking though his options as he formed his next sentence.

"They're going to keep asking," he said, waving the letters. "You know that's why they sent you the plate. They thought you'd joined the church and give them money."

"They said it was free. They can't make me."

"Nope. They cannot."

I straightened my plate. Dad turned to leave.

I looked at my altar. It was nice enough, but the closet was a little dusty, and I didn't fit in it with the door closed. Not comfortably. And despite at least a week of devotion, no hand of love lifted me out of that which I had not chosen, and could not bear, and dropped me back at the Nubble.

I thought about my occasional playmate who lived across the road from our last house in Massachusetts. Scotty Winslow was a born anarchist and fire-eater. On a summer day, after much back and forthing with me about how "he wouldn't dare/oh yes he would", he'd said "there's no such thing as God" *out loud*. I'd shivered. Looked to the sky. Waited to record the moment of his being lightning-struck, since that was the only way this was going to go.

And yet, no. It was a warm blue day and the Yankee trees around us shivered with contentment in the sun. Un-smitten Scotty was grinning to hide his own relief. Was it possible, I thought for the first time, that the god I'd heard promoted on the Sundays Teen took me to church was not all that was advertised?

Oral, the lying minister who offered free to the faithful and then demanded gold, was now adding to that doubt. A moment later came the third and conclusive blow to my life among the faithful.

My Dad turned back as he was leaving my room, looked at my plate and the letters ranting about the potential collapse of civilization if I didn't send Oral some seed. His father-knows-best straight face flat out failed him before he could get out of my room, and he broke. Laughter wheezed out of him as he moved quickly down the hall.

That was it. Anything my father thought was ridiculous wasn't going to work for me. Mom and I getting off on the wrong foot was becoming something made of stone. Teen was miles and miles away, and increasingly, I was being told that to harp on going back to her was stupid and histrionic, so I'd best give that up. I couldn't afford to lose Dad too. Among other things, he was the only one I could see driving me back to New England.

Fortunately I had a huge moon snail shell that Teen gave me. "Hold it to your ear honey," she'd said, "and you can hear the ocean." I pushed the stuff in the chapel to the back of the closet, and looked at the shell. Oh that's silly, I thought, the ocean can't fit in there. But, still, I walked over, picked it up and put the great white thing to my ear.

And there it was; the rushing thud of the surf, real as the hand of God wasn't. The big ocean, in my ear. And I, its child, though at a great distance, waiting. Just waiting. But with faith.

I would grow up. I would figure it out. I would get back to the lighthouse.

Leaving America 2017

And Eric says he'll get me to Maine. Weird, dubious, but for the moment it seems that's not going to be how this trip gets taken away from me. So I shift all my considerable capacity for worry to whether I will get through U.S. customs.

This trip will be my first border crossing since I renounced my American citizenship. Trump had since taken America—and now I am not sure they will let me back in.

I went a little crazy when they elected Trump. By crazy I mean, on Twitter, all day, every day, most nights, for, oh, six months. Looking for the announcement. That they knew it was rigged. That it was all set aside. That this Paddy Chayefsky version of my former country was going to melt away, like snagged film, bubbling and sizzling and finally flapping into white light. As if it never was. Because it couldn't be.

'Because he was a joke, eh? Pathetic. Absurd. An obscene, posturing, childishly self-aggrandizing clown from some heavy-handed expressionist play, soiling his bulbous pants, and kicking his oversized booties in theatrical tantrums. A cartoon villain. Bugs Bunny was supposed to waltz in, lay a big fat wet one on him, and shove him in the corner, with an exploding cigar in his mouth.

He was Doh-Doh the Dirty Clown, and you wouldn't buy a used car from him.[17]

But instead, there seemed to be people in America who absolutely relished life with Doh-Doh. All the things they wanted to do but couldn't because they were now considered "bad," Doh-Doh had already done. Hate. Grab. Take. Leave his engine running as he ate endangered rhinos off plastic plates in Antarctica while watching Putin's gift-with-purchase prostitutes pee on beds of shredded civil rights.

Doh-Doh did that. So they could too.

I obsessively read stories about the expanding powers and boldness of customs officials. Pussy hat wearing protesters sent home. Cell phone histories read and owners banned. ICE and IRS on speed dial. America seemed to see my Canadian citizenship as an act of treason when I was dealing with the minions of Bush Jr. This time, I have not only said yes to Canada, I've said piss-off to the U.S.

I think they are going to put me in jail.

Strip searches, missed connections and days at the embassy in Boston trying to get in is clearly in my future. I play the mental tape of being pulled out of the line, walked to a room, not allowed to speak to Eric. Like most of my overly-sensitive, nut job visions, it is the worst of many possible outcomes, but entirely plausible.

I talk with a friend who comes from a town not far from where I was born. He simply no longer crosses the border.

"What does it say on your passport?" he asks.

"Born in Gardner, Massachusetts."

He looks puzzled for a minute.

"Westminster was too small for a hospital."

"Well, you're fucked."

I look at Eric in triumph—I love it when my crazy gets corroborated. Eric gives our friend a baleful I-could-strangle-you-with-my-bare-

---

17. I wrote this section before the children in cages. The pandemic. The armed insurrection. Imagine what I would write now.

hands-and-that-would-stillnot-undo-the-harm-you've-just-done-but-ooooo-would-it-feel-good look. Says, "I think you are making yourself anxious over what will be a non-issue."

So what? I'm good at that. And besides I have rock solid evidence to support this latest bout of nutty. It has already happened.

I am sitting looking at an unsatisfactory lunch. I am under armed guard. I have snatched a few moments conversation with Eric, who has been waiting for me for four hours without being permitted to sit. There are no chairs, and he was told to get off the floor when he tried to rest. Summer of 2013 was weird and full of flood and we are both dragged out with humidity, the long drive from Regina to Calgary, bad sleep, and unexpressed rage. I am also still partly covered in mud.

I tell him to go. It will be hours, and I will go and get my things and call him when I am free. My bag with wallet and phone are in a $15 lock-up at the YMCA, ten blocks and a stumble through what turned out to be a construction site (which I only learned when the crane operator began to scream at me, and I started to run, thick Alberta clay ruining my shoes and stockings) away.

He goes and I stare at the plate. I cannot swallow the food. I have been fighting sobbing for hours and it sticks in my throat.

I am not in jail, I am at my embassy, the American Embassy, in Calgary, Alberta. I am trying to leave America. And they will not let me.

"You will walk in a single line. You will enter the elevator in groups of six. If you move from your group, you will be taken from the building."

Five hours earlier, I am staring at the kid guarding us. He must be Canadian, right? I mean they wouldn't pay an American kid to move to guard what has to be the safest American embassy in the world.

If he's not American, he is *taking* to it. What did they do? Give him a gun and a laminated card to keep in his rent-a-cop breast pocket that says:

Always act like you want to shoot someone.

Always talk louder than necessary.

Always be mean to brown people.

Because that's who most of us are—some sixty mostly brown people who want to get into America. And me, who wants to get out. The others are of every age from pram riders to impossibly old, dried wood figures that creak with every step. There are turbans and saris and burkas and kurtas and dashikis. There is language and culture and colour, all squashed under that voice. That mean. That gun.

"Your hands will be visible. At all times."

I assume the "I Will Fuck You Up" stance is on the back of the laminated card.

I try to talk to him cheerfully, I'm-old-enough-to-be-your-mom-fully. Remind him who he is. That this is a bad dream. Outside, it's still Calgary, and Stampede is just over and young things with flowers in the bands of their cowboy hats are sipping soy lattes, figuring out what to pack for the Folk Festival.

Nothing. The fear of the other and the faith in the gun have already gone so deep in this kid that were he a dog, I would run. This one will bite.

I name him Young Gun. He'll be our designated shouter today.

Between the shouting and the very formal language, a number of people do not seem to understand what they are supposed to do. Young Gun shouts louder. I think I should intervene, but I too am afraid. I settle for using the astonished look usually reserved for those who talk during movies on Young Gun, and a warm smile and a slow and clear explanation of the instructions for the small, sharp-featured man who looks like he comes from Eritrea maybe (?).

Up the lift and then a forced march into a long beige room, split down the middle by panes of thick yellowish, bullet (and probably bomb proof) glass. Behind the panes are middle-aged, blank-faced, wary white people wearing summer white people clothes. We are shouted at to take numbers, because clearly no one here has seen *Beetlejuice*, or, if they have, they don't know it's supposed to be funny. "Sit and wait for your number to be called." Not a problem for me. I'm alone with fifteen chairs right under the big flag on the American side of a velvet rope. The people on the other side of the rope also have fifteen chairs. For sixty of them. This is a problem, and the ones left standing look frightened.

I'm also still frightened. I am nothing but frightened. This entire process has been turning my sleep to sweat and starts, and my bowels to fiery water for more than a year. But the fifteen chairs and being on the *right* side of the rope are settling my nerves a bit. My number is called first. Up I go to a narrow opening in the yellow glass.

"I have come to renounce my American citizenship," holding my papers out to a 40-ish civil servant, long, hippie-plaited hair, soft western accent, maybe Wyoming, wearing the kind of sweater that women who infinitely prefer cats to well…just about anything, favour. She looks appalled.

"Leave those with us," not touching the offending pieces of paper, "You can come back in six to eight weeks."

"What? No. I talked to the embassy in Toronto." The embassy in Calgary does not answer the phone. The embassy in Calgary does not have a phone. The embassy in Calgary is in some kind of witness protection program. "They said if I had all the documents in place I could come here and renounce today."

"Yes. We have a different protocol than Toronto."

"Which is?"

"We like to allow for a cooling off period."

"Pardon me?"

"Sugar, once you calm down, we both know you'll change your mind."

I look at her. She goes pale. So you know how I look at her.

My panic-and-procrastinate response since deciding to renounce has been so severe that, rather than fill in the damn documents required for the process all at once, I developed an incremental approach. Day One, I sharpen a pencil. Put it on my desk and assume the recovery position under my desk before the hyperventilation makes me black out. Day Two, I give the pencil an eraser to keep it company and crawl away. Day Three, I read a page and make a list of things I must do. Vomit. Think I should read another. Do not. It has taken a year, but every single year of my life in Canada, four decades and change, is documented. I am good with the tax man. I can see the light. And now this.

I like to think of myself as all Canadian. I try to be all-Canadian. But now something *older* burbles up.

"Yes. *Sugar?* I drove nine hours from Regina with a special needs teenager to get here. I am not doing that again. I am plenty calm. I want to renounce today."

She looks at me.

"Well … there're things I have to check. I'll try to call some people. See if we can get this through. It'll take a while — "

"— great. Can I pay the fee now? So it's done?"

Sugar looks hurt. Oh. She was going to try, sort of. Not hard enough that she wanted to take my money. I clench my wallet, and walk over to the wicket where there's a till. Look back to her.

"I am really not going to leave until I renounce."

A few moments and four hundred dollars later, I sit down, performatively. And realize that I am now being watched. Not just by Sugar, who is looking at me like I ate one of her kittens, but by Young Gun, who has strolled closer, assuming a position of authority under the Stars and Bars, and by a sweaty, self-important man I can see through the glass. He has been alternating between glaring at my paperwork, reaming Sugar out, and staring at me, as one would stare at some kind of aberration. Y'know. A two-headed goat. Dog-faced boy. American who wants out. After a while though, everyone seems to settle down and get back to the normal and expected business of the day, which is keeping the sixty other people who (properly) want in, out.

You see, there are two Americas. I mean there's thousands, but if concepts of nationhood were hotels, people from the thousands of Americas would stay at one of two chains:

There's the Jeffersonian America Inn. It was invented by a bunch of frat boys through a sweaty summer in the middle of a war about money who espoused the inalienable rights of, well, initially landed white men, and backed it with a system for free elections and the unbiased enforcement of law. That's where me and mine would stay.

Then there's the other one. The America Uber Alles Palace, where White is Right, and that's ours, that's also ours, and that's ours too; and no you can't come in and have ANY of it, and if you try we'll *shoot* you. And yes we can, 'cause we're *America*, bitches. You know, the psycho one?

The people with no chairs? That's who they're dealing with.

I grew up constantly reminded that I was a descendant of presidents (the connection between my branch of the Adams family and the two Adams presidents is not quite as close as my family insists, but still). Democracy and freedom and the idea of equality were invented where I come from—and that matters. I memorised the Declaration of Independence. I studied the Constitution. I can sing every song from the musical 1776. At this moment, it seems that, despite my fear, I have an obligation to represent for our team.

A woman on the wrong side of the rope shifts from one foot to another, adjusts her sari. She's very old. And has been standing for more than an hour because her husband needs to sit more.

I make an offer.

"Ma'am, would you like my chair?"

"Those seats are for American citizens only." This is from Young Gun.

"It's only the chair I would be using. I'll stand. Do you want me to move it to the other side of the rope?"

"Whatever."

Overheard at the open wicket:

"You-need-a-witness-for-this-sale-to-go-through," this is delivered as one irrefutable word (for, no doubt, the thousandth time) by an embassy staffer.

"I've been here three hours already. No one never told me I had to get a witness."

"Well you do."

Offer.

"I can be his witness," smiling ear to ear at the face behind the glass. Sign everything put in front of me (quite possibly the purchase of Florida swampland) with a flourish. I go to the washroom and clear the construction mud from my legs and throw my stockings in the garbage. I wash my face. Go back out and stand on the fortunate side of the rope.

There are terribly bored children running up and down the room in mindless laps, passing ever closer to Young Gun. He twitches, and when one 5-year-old potential terrorist gets too close, places his hand on his holster. I can already hear the evening news: "The guard said his training just kicked in, 'Kids with bombs are part of what we train for, and hesitating to shoot can result in more lives lost.'"

Again.

"Kids? Kids? You want a story? C'mere. Once upon a time, there was a monkey (my squeaky voice) and a shark (my growl) ..." They have no idea what I'm saying but the funny voices seem to go over, and they stop running and don't become the lead story on CBC Calgary.

I make an offer to the people on the wrong side of the rope. A counter-offer to the people behind the glass. A *suggestion* to Young Gun. I walk crying babies, help elderly women to the washroom, and escort one person after another to *my* chair on which I have planted my flag and freedom reigns. I am the star-spangled, maple leaf-covered Mary Poppins of being *decent* in a beige room. And I am having the time of my life.

"Kelley Burke?"

I bounce over to Sugar's wicket. She's been on the phone for hours. Calling who? Well, the Government of Canada to check that I am truthfully one of theirs. Social Security, to confirm the number that I have only just acquired at the U.S. government's insistence and have to give back, in order to renounce, is for real, probably. The IRS to make sure I am cleared up with them. Homeland Security? Because I see the symbol for it on her computer screen. She did say something about having to do a criminal record check when she was trying to put me off (wouldn't you think they'd *want* to see the back of me if I was a bad apple?). She gives me a steady look.

"Having fun?"

I smile.

"Everyone is going for lunch. We're going to send you downstairs to get something to eat, and when you come back, this'll all be done."

Great.

I go down the elevator with Young Gun, who stands armed guard over me as I eat, lest I commit an act of terror with my hummus. And then I see her. Sugar. She has a coat and a brief case and she is slipping down the stairwell and out the building. Head turned. Avoiding my questioning face. She doesn't look like someone going for lunch. She looks like someone calling it a day. And then I see another person from behind the yellow glass. Same. And another.

The blood rushes to my head and feet simultaneously and I am speaking well before I have fully processed what I have just seen. I can only be grateful that I taught high school and Young Gun attended one.

"Take me back upstairs. *Right now.*"

It comes out pure, chalk-covered Grade 11 English teacher. That apparently trumps the gun.

Sure enough, when we get upstairs the beige room is empty. All the other applicants are gone (I don't know *what* they did with them). The wicket people are putting their chairs on their desks, calling it a day. The sweaty man is exiting stage right as fast as ever he can. I stand, watch and then—

Excuse me?"

Busted. I don't have to tell him who I am. He doesn't tell me. Or that this let's-send-her-for-lunch-and-don't-tell-her-that's-when-we-close-until-it's-too-late move is his. We have not spoken directly yet, but we have been speaking *at* each other all day. He is the Deputy U.S. Consul. I am the Disloyal Opposition.

"I am renouncing today."

He takes a huge breath. Looks braced to argue. I slap down my receipt.

"I've already paid."

His shoulders fall. He hands me another form, and it is surprisingly brief. I fill it in quickly, then think better and slow down. Don't make a mistake; they will use it to punt the whole thing. Quite possibly make me re-immigrate. I hand back the completed form and take up a final single sheet of paper with the oath that I must swear in answer to his questions, printed out.

"Raise your right h—," he stops.

"What?"

He sits back, tilts his head to one side, takes a moment and then leans in.

"Have you thought about this?"

My jaw drops, Looney Tune' style. I say none of the things that spring to mind. None. I'm too close to indulge in outrage at this point. Instead:

"Well. I've been in Canada since I was six. I've been a Canadian since I was twenty-one. I've been *here* all day. So. Yes. I have *thought* about this."

His face is flushed, almost teary. I realize what I'm looking at is grief. For me. And sheer incomprehension that one of *us* would throw away what so many of *them* would die for.

Raise my right hand and read, looking up and meeting his eyes with the end of every line:

I desire and hereby make a formal renunciation of my U.S. nationality, as provided by section 349(a)(5) of the Immigration and Nationality Act of 1952, as amended, and pursuant thereto, I hereby absolutely and entirely renounce my United States nationality together with all rights and privileges and all duties and allegiance and fidelity thereunto pertaining. I make this renunciation intentionally, voluntarily, and of my own free will, free of any duress or undue influence.

It is formal and ritualized, like something from a black and white movie, done by men in flannel suits. It is very, very American.

And let's face it, so am I. But not like that. Never like that. Please.

One more offer. Perhaps someone can be saved.

"Hey? Young Gun?"

Young Gun looks confused and tries to assume the stance.

"What?"

I hold arms out wide enough to hold him, if necessary, carry him. I beam.

"C'mon. Let's get the fuck out of here."

I realize, trying to visualize this first trip to America after forcing them to let me go, that *this* will be the evil angels' play to take the lighthouse away again. They will dress like U.S. Customs. Stare at my offensive passport. Pull me away from the kiosk. Tell me I have to walk to a beige room without windows. They will put their hands on their holsters as they make Eric leave, without speaking to me. I will sit there. For hours. Explaining again and again why I renounced. There are mistakes that I can make in my answers that will make my renunciation illegal. The angels know that. They know I will trip up.

As our plane goes. And our deposit goes, Gabrielle shaking her head, wondering why, after all her good gifts to me, I have failed to get to her. And I will never get in.

I never think of being back at the lighthouse as being back in America. The thought of getting so close to the Nubble only to be blocked by the country that happens to hold it is so painful I cannot breathe.

The angels shuffle on their perches, bat their wings, and prepare to strike.

The Money 1996

Later, on the night of the whales, I walk into the Anchorage Hotel. There is blood on my hands, a rip in my dress, and a crab claw in my hair. The desk clerk doesn't blink. Clearly off-season people walk in from worse dates in York Beach, Maine.

I turn the light out in my hotel room and open the screen door. Listen. Long Sands Beach is right across the street. I can't see the waves coming in, because, as predicted, the fog is now a soft white wall. I can't see the Nubble either, not even the red eye, but I hear it, the fog horn lowing the warning that began as I'd crawled away from my whale-in-the-water adventure.

I look down at my bleeding palms. The room starts to spin and I sit hard on the bed. I am having a so-*that*-happened moment. They tend to be quite physical. Electric bolts dance at the edge of my eyes. Uh oh.

Start the calming process; three deep breaths, centre and imagine myself safe on my rock. Usually when I do this, I am thousands of miles away. Tonight I have just left where I sit in my imagination. This starts me spinning again.

A tickle in my stomach. I think of the last whale scraping into the water, of my own painful stumbling back from what I discovered was the brink, when my shoes began taking water. Crazy...

Giggling. Would like to tell someone. Would like to believe getting at least one whale in the water has laid Teen's ghost. Bought her peace. Something. Would like, I notice, swaying in rhythm with the surf sounds, to be having sex, like right now. The pound of the tide makes that more acute.[18]

Think to earlier in this day, when, trying to calm down after a few hours in the cottage, I'd been on the beach. The thick brown sludge of Liquid Gold and dust grief was coating my mouth, lungs, belly—closing my throat. So I went to Long Sands to wash it out. Stood at the edge. Let the surf sound close around me. Not enough, Too far away. Did not decide. Simply, and despite the lateness of the season and the cold that is always the North Atlantic, walked fully clothed into the rough surf. The buffeting and roar briefly enough to carry me out of what I'd left behind.

To my left, I saw a man doing *exactly* the same thing. Up to his armpits. Dressed. Taking the waves' beating like expiation. I'd passed him earlier, as I parked and headed down to the beach. He was the driver of a van for high needs kids. By the look of the restraints and tanks I could see inside, the van's passengers were very high need. Watching him stare out as he was battered by the cold sea, it seemed to me that there was no one else in the world now but us. That if I waded through the surf to him, he would not be surprised. He would hold out his arms, and press my face to his chest, arms warm around my spray-soaked shirt, and say, "Finally."

Half of me was already doing this.

Fortunately, on *many* levels, including not yet having an arrest record in the state of Maine and hoping to keep it that way, I resisted. Stayed in my section of the surf. Watched him head safely, soggily, back to his van.

But I need sex now. I want a big finish, to consecrate the burial

---

18. It's the euphoria. When you are very anxious and think you are going to die all the time, and then you don't, you get a lot of post near-death euphoria, which adds a nice, unhinged, swinging-from-the-chandelier top note to your base panicked-nutsy.

at sea I've conducted on the rocks. Celebrate living to tell the tale. I want to catch a champagne fount of my salt water in cupped hands, leave some fantasy lover gaping on the questionable bed and run naked out of the hotel to the surf. Pour myself into the greater sea, like some boutique religion priestess. Stomp and storm and howl. Let sand scour my nethers[19] free of the yellow, stinking sadness clinging to them.

Realizing this would also be a crime and leave me open to comments at the breakfast buffet tomorrow, I try to bring my mind back to the crime I *have* committed. I have stolen Grampa's financial records: his will, his investment documents, the titles to the property. I'm trying to figure out what he can afford for help. The print is hard to make out, the hotel room not as well-lit as it might be. The Anchorage is getting a little rundown. But it is clean, sort of, and opens to the beach, and for that I would sleep on a float mattress on the hotel lawn. I have all the windows wide. Gulp the cold air. Better.

I scoured the cottage. Broke into the safe. Rifled the drawers of the roll top writing desk in his bedroom. While my grandfather slept in the chair, dreaming of the brown-skinned wrackers whom he expects in the night, come to steal the silver that Teen has long since sewed into the back of the sofa, and so no joy for them, I had done much worse.

I moved by the dim light, which will figure repeatedly in my dreams yet to come. Teeth clenched, quiet but defiant, I stuffed the pertinent papers, secret agent style, into my trench coat. Fled here.

The documents affirm a couple of things. One that I still come from money. Or at least I come halfway from money, on Mom's side. The money that comes from land, held and added to and accrued over hundreds of years in Westminster, Mass. Turned to dollars when Grampa sold Adams Street, and all the other holdings in Westminster, and my great-grandmother's stocks (she bought IBM at

---

19. At its worst, this is where the euphoria leads. The reckless and gratuitous use of the word "nethers."

something like eight), winterized the cottage at the Nubble and left Massachusetts a well-to-do man, which is to say, in America, a man armoured. Cased in stone.

Coming from money is everything in America. It is class. It is worth. It is freedom from fear. It is what Mom was prepared to walk from, theoretically, when she got knocked up by Dad. Dad didn't have money, not even a little, which is why he should *not* have inseminated my mother. The constant threat that the whole family lived under was that the Adams money would never be ours if things got so bad between my parents and Mom's dad that Grampa cut her out of the will.

When that was mentioned, my dad would bark, "Let him." He was the new order; a poor Irish-trash boy who was educated. Jumped right into a white collar. A professor with tenure and a tweed jacket with leather elbow patches and a G-D pipe. The money, and anyone attached to it who still thought that old silver trumped reinvention, could go to hell and he'd call them a cab.

Except. Except.

After nine years teaching in Canada, Dad got sick. Really sick. We were on sabbatical in Edmonton.[20] My dad longed to be one of those guys, the guys who don't make the rent but make wealth, who play deep at the blackjack table, who sit in the owner's box, sipping imported beer, smiling the smile of well-fed sharks, one to each. So he gambled on selling our house in Winnipeg and buying another in Edmonton and then rolling it. The equity in our Winnipeg place was everything we had, but good fellows, decent sorts, promised Dad that with the 1975/6 real estate market in Edmonton he would rise up out of it with the kind of money that always eluded him. Instead he dropped. On the floor, in a grand mal seizure, breaking furniture, blood from the sides of his chewed tongue turning his spittle pink and frothy.

---

20. My friends, also all children of academics, went to India for sabbaticals, where they had servants, and cobras in the garden. Or Fiji, where they dove for pink pearls. Japan. Mexico. Wales. We went to Edmonton.

He came home from the hospital alone. Walked in and said to his three kids, the youngest eight years old, "There is a tumour in my brain. They can't remove it. Because of where it is. If they try, it'll make me a vegetable ..." Except partway through the "vegetable" he broke, all two-hundred and fifty plus pounds of him, melting into high-pitched wheezing and sobs that could not be the product of my father but rather of some heart broken and abandoned beast. That's when my mother walked in.

One look, and she had the entire situation, the sobbing man, and the staggered children watching, pupils dilated. The question of breaking down and joining her husband in showing their collective underbelly to the children was not considered. Instead, a military precision. A snap and the kids were moved to the rec room (absolutely no objections there — we would have cut and run earlier except the universe ended right in front of us and we didn't remember how to do feet). Snap again. Dad was in my parents' bedroom, still keening, the sound horrible and persistent under the door. Mom's face was that of someone ready to murder either the weeping heap inside, or anyone who so much as *looked wrong* at the weeping heap inside.

And then Dad wasn't about the collar or the jacket or the pipe. Dad was about the tumour. And about the money that we wouldn't have once the tumour killed Dad.

The roll-a-house thing went bust. We lost every cent of equity from the sale of our Winnipeg house, trying to unload the Edmonton one. Mom worked, but it wasn't enough to keep a roof over three kids, and who knew how much longer Dad had?

It was awful. We kids didn't know how awful, but once in a while we'd get a snapshot. Mom leaning into our whining for her to buy one thing or another, hissing "we can't afford *ketchup*." Dad slipping me some cash and murmuring into his beard, "Maybe don't tell your mom." Snippets of their conversations:

"He has to help."

"I don't know that he does."

"Who has to help?"

"Kelley, this is an adult conversation."

"But you said —"

"This is not your business."

The state of our finances, why we were now renting an ugly little bungalow in the white trash/single parent/grad student/support staff section of our old neighborhood was mostly understood through the quality of the air in the house. Every breath was taut, costly, as if some lugubrious heavy metal was transformed into gas, and we were supposed to suck it up. Dad spent hours sitting in a chair in the basement, not sleeping, not talking. Holding his head as if careful cradling would win the tumour's forgiveness, stop the endless and exhausting seizures.

He had to ask Grampa for money.

All Dad would ever say about that, and this was well after my grandfather was dead, was, "I was dying. You guys were all still kids. And he was calling around for prime rates and compound interest plans to write up and have me sign." And then he'd bow his now scarred head, saved by an experimental surgery, the triangular bit of radiation-scored skin covering his never-healing, hinged chunk of skull, a once and future doorway to his brain.

That's what the Money was. To be there, untouched and shining, for the moment when Reinvention faltered, and Old Money, that was shaken by the New Deal-civil rights-leveled-playing-field democracy nonsense of recent days, could once more hold these truths to be self-evident

1. A college degree can't buy you the right bones in the graveyard.
2. The inferior are inferior because their lack of breeding leaves them weak in purpose, foolish in practice, and exactly where they belong.
3. Anyone who thinks different is goddamn stupid.

What else could Dad do? The tumour was breaking all of us — Mom seemed to put everything she felt into a single blue-white blaze of rage that wanted nothing but a target — but which one was always up for grabs. I was ticking though a list of things designed to get a teenage girl pregnant, jailed, or dead, though not necessarily in that order. Brother Steve in the back of police cars or the back of stores, holding to his terrified chimp grin as he was grilled for one petty crime or another. Sister Jess, now nine, simply watching, unsurprised, as we fell apart.

He signed the papers Grampa sent him. We bought a house exactly like our old house on a better lot. We moved in. Waited for Dad to die. And gave the Money the day.

In a secret corner of my mind, I still took quiet guilty comfort in the Money. Teen always said if I wanted to come live with her, I could. The Money could make that happen. It would not treat me as it treated my father, not Kelley living in Canada like a tourist, clutching her return ticket for home. The Money wanted me back.

Which was good because things were still terrible. Dad was working, but heavily drugged, and, despite the drugs, wracked by petit mal seizures and often slurred and confused. Campus rumour was that he was a drunk. At seventeen, my job was to sit up with him after my mother went to bed and talk about that, for hours, and about his pain and fear and coming death.[21] To receive that which my mother, far less able to endure such conversations, would not. Which made me feel very grownup. And special. And like a sadness bomb ripe to explode. Also, in my dealings with Mom, smug. Which made things much more terrible.

What could I do but think of the Money?

I could call my grandparents. I could run out … on all of them. The lighthouse was waiting. Not sick. Not sad. Ready and firm. That was keeping me alive.

Except.

It came. The moment. Mom and I went at it, again, me sobbing so hard I seemed to be wrenching inside out. Her words coming like the rush from a crumbling dam: I was a fat, self-indulgent, self-important, interfering idiot, who, in the face of a dying father and

---

21. Yes, I was much too young. And yes, he was a psychologist and knew better. I think I'd need to carry a time bomb in my skull for a while before I got to be too judgey about that.

a mother who just needed someone to do as she was told, kept insisting on *herself*.

I finally choked out, "If it's so bad having me here, send me to Teen."

My mother almost smiled, "Oh no. We talked. They don't want you either."

I stood there, in our bilious paisley 70s rec room, red-faced under buzzing fluorescents. Thought: Well. No. Of course they don't. I am those things she said, and nothing like the girl my grandparents loved, white-dressed and sweet. Nothing like a keeper's daughter. Of course they don't want me.

The Money wasn't there for me. And it wasn't (as it turned out) for Teen, either.

The last time I saw my grandmother alive, it seemed insane to leave her in the cottage. After a lifetime of mixing downers and booze, she was not competent. The cellar stairs were a broken hip waiting to happen. The food in the fridge suspect. The stove was left on high for hours ... every day. And not a fire alarm in sight.

I had two children of my own at that point, and would not bring them into a cottage full of loaded guns and red hot elements. We rented up the hill, and when I came down Nubble Road to see her, sometimes she knew me, sometimes not. This speech played like a looped tape several times a day:

"We are so happy here."

"I know Teen."

"We had to take care of Jim's (my grandfather's) old people back in Westminster ... We could never be here as much as we wanted."

"I know, Teen."

"But now it is so good here."

"Well. Yes."

So she wasn't safe. But she was, when in her loop, happy. And there was plenty of money. To pay for the hospital when she needed it. To pay for someone to come in and make sure she didn't take too many pills, again. Someone to keep her safe. If someone had forced the old man to spend it, by a court order if necessary. If someone believed even for a minute that money could be something other than preservation of class. Worth. Freedom from fear. If any of us tried even a little to make it be something else. But none of us did.

"She's going to burn the house down," I told my mom after that last time with Teen.

"There are worse ways for old people to die."

The papers stop making sense. An hour with them has pretty much killed my euphoria. I shuffle them away and think how I will put them back tomorrow without being seen.

Mom will get the Money. When the total comes in, my still-not-dead father will look at my mother and ask, "So, are you leaving me now?" And it will stop being a joke somewhere around the last word.

I come from money. But the Money was never about me. Trusting the money was a chump's game, like God, or hanging my hat on the love of a husband who belonged to someone else, or random sex with strangers in the sea. None of these things will give me what I need.

What I need is stepping out from the fog now. I see her red eye winking. I lean into the balcony railing, and breathe in wisps of vapour that carry the lighthouse's scent.

The Burkes 2018

I look out the door at Auntie Pam's side porch.

"Oh Pam."

"I know."

"Salmon."

"I know."

"Salmon Pink?"

"I went everywhere. All over town. No one had the right —"

"Ballerina Pink, Pam. Has to be *Ballerina* Pink."

"I don't know what she'd say."

Yes she does. We both do.

We are staying with my Burke family in New Hampshire for the couple of days before we can get into the cottage in Maine. It's Memorial Day and my Auntie Pam and I are surveying the flowers she bought to plant on my *other* grandmother's grave.

(Going through Customs earlier that day was of course nothing. We entered the U.S. through the gate at the Ottawa airport. I approached. A woman looked at my passport. Asked me about my trip. Asked where Eric was. I pointed behind me — I was so nervous I bolted to the post, wanting to get it over with. She said something lovely and southern-flavoured about me having a good time, and it was over. I walked up an incline, rolling my suitcase. The sound of Eric's completely silent, resolutely unvoiced, freakin' *mute* "I told you so" was so loud my ears bled a little.)

Anyway, we'd made it to the Burke family compound in Penacook: a broad, white, sagging old house, divided into two mostly separate homes, with a front porch wrapped around both and a 200-plus-year-old barn that stands behind, out of habit and in defiance of gravity. There are pokey stairways, narrow rooms and endless things that need to be repaired, because nobody said being authentically Yankee was supposed to be fun. Almost everyone in my New Hampshire Burke family has lived in some part of it, at some time.

I make it sound like I only have one place, one family, to go home to. Of course I have two: the Adams, and the one from which I take my name, the Burkes. And the Burkes are a whole other kettle of Friday fish.

The Adams are landed, moneyed, arch-conservative, tight-lipped, tighter-fisted and heavily armed. They aren't beholden to anyone. Never buy what they can make. Never throw away what can be used again. They have land not cash. Name not fame. Wear their whiteness like a medal, sink their gnarled roots, deeper than the deepest trees into the spare, rocky Massachusetts soil, and chant "MINE" to the crisp autumn air. You know ... Protestants.

The *Burkes* are immigrant Irish, three generations back, and they're still sorry about it. There is a bend to the shoulder and an apology for taking up space you get with a Burke that I think comes from the time when Irish meant dirty, plague-ridden, and criminal, the unwanted, unwashed that the Adams of the past thought we shouldn't be harbouring until "our own are looked after." When that's where you come from, it behooves you to withhold judgement. Vote Democrat. Work in helping professions. Eat heartily when you have it. Share even when you don't. Drink until it's gone. Light up because you're going to die anyhow. Laugh at anything, the darker the better. Weep in public. Sing while laughing and weeping—

in public. You know. Catholics.[22]

And being with the Burkes is just ... a joy. The joy of shared history and genetics and picking up the conversation exactly where you left off, though you left it ten years before. I *love* it. I love them. Which begs the question, why do I not pine to come home to that? Why, instead, do I have this spawning salmon's thrash-panic need to get to a lighthouse to which I have no claim? A panic which is obvious, and I suspect hurtful as I sit in Pam's kitchen.

We don't talk about that. But we talk about everything else. The living. The dead. Mostly the dead. And what my Grandmother Burke would say about salmon pink geraniums.

Gramma wouldn't spit on Pam's flowers or anything. She'd sigh a little, her tongue resting on her lower lip. Cross to the coffee pot, all five foot nothin' of her, and somewhat spherical, though absolutely form-fitted by terrifying neck to ankle girdles that hung like headless and exsanguinated Bluebeard's wives from sateen-pillowed hangers in her closet, with the rolling stride of someone who by the end could not walk in anything but high heels, because her feet were fused into an arch. Pour herself another cup. Look about for something sweet to go with it. Wonder out loud if maybe somebody might go look again. For the right colour of geraniums. Somehow hint that someone better than Pam could certainly find them.

Gramma wanted things pretty. Ballerina pretty. And life did not hand her that. So armoured in modestly priced, tightly coordinated business dresses, hair so spray-shellacked with White Rain that it did not move in the strongest wind, and pungent with a tragic addiction to Avon cologne (Cotillion in the Ballerina Pink bottle, Moonwind in the Princess Blue), she worked with what she had: a functional alcoholic husband on the night shift and two sons on emotional tenterhooks. But when Son Number One ran off with his family to Canada and my Grandfather Burke died, Gramma had to move in with her (not faithless and abandoning) Son Number Two

---

22. Though these days they're mostly Episcopalian, i.e. Catholic-lite. All the candles, half the guilt.

(my lovely Uncle Jeff), and his (inadequate in Gramma's opinion) wife, Pam. And it became my aunt's job to keep things Ballerina Pink for Dorothy Burke. Until she died.

"... I went to the hospital to give her something ... She was crying and said, "Why are you so good to me? And I'm awful to you." I told her "Dot, you're my mother-in-law. I love you ..." and I meant it and I was glad to do it. But it was ... what I mean to say is ... I understand, now, why your parents decided to move away."

Each time I visit Penacook, Pam forgives me for my part in my family's leaving her behind with all that care. It has nothing to do with failing memory. Pam is a (great) teacher, and she never repeats things without intention. She is modelling a conscious decision to let resentments go. Like how long she tried to keep things pretty for Dorothy Burke. How much time that took from the total number of years she had with my (adored and adoring) Uncle Jeff, before he died in her arms.

But, if she can let her past griefs go, says Pam the teacher with her eyes, shouldn't I? My obsession with being taken from the lighthouse might be a place to start.

Then she adds aloud, "I know you have had more tragedy than most."

We don't go into the list. Dad's illness. Teen's sort-of murder. Accidents of birth and violations of spirit.

Steve.

My brother Steve dropped dead on a Tuesday afternoon in January 2005. He got up from his desk in the rec room of my parents' house where he lived, and crossed to the bathroom. Dropped and died, halfway there.

Eric answered our phone in Regina. I looked up. His voice was odd, as if he was trying to catch up with what he was being told and could not think what sound to make. He said something to me and held out the phone. It sounded like "Steve has died."

My mother found him at the foot of the basement stairs. There were flashing lights and sirens, paramedics and futility.

"He was so cold," my mother said.

I told her I would come right away. I tried to walk upstairs to pack. My first in-focus memory is of the purple nap of the rug on our stairs. I got to the second step and then was face down, wide-eyed, screaming, "Get up. Get off the fucking rug. Save baby brother Steve." The screaming made no sound.

Did Eric find me there? I don't think so. I think he was calling to get me a compassionate flight to Winnipeg. Realized I had to tell my kids, who adored my brother. Got up. Did that. Like a training video for parents doing grief with their kids. Said things. Said we loved them. Over and over. But there's little memory there either, except the look of pure rage on my son Sam's face.

And so to Winnipeg. And Trying to Help. I worked as a producer for the CBC in January of 2005, so since "I" remained on the rug in Regina, unable to stop screaming, I asked Producer Kelley Jo to take the wheel. And she was game. Put on her Ballerina Pink hat and welcomed the friends who came to support her absolutely devastated parents. Catalogued the casseroles delivered and who owned what dish. Decided how many chairs to put out for the memorial, how many flowers, that the ash box should have a monogram of a guitar above Steve's name. And it was she who wrote his obituary:

> It is with deep sadness that we announce the death of Stephen James Burke. He died unexpectedly, and without suffering, at his home, on January 25, 2005 at 40 years of age, of an aortic aneurism... Stephen was a gifted man. But his greatest gift was for friendship. Affectionate, funny and incredibly loyal, Steve had the ability not only to make friends but to hold onto them, through life changes and distance and time ...

On the "Affectionate, funny and incredibly loyal" line, the person back on the rug in Regina showed up briefly. Producer Kelley Jo (PKJ) got hold of her, and finished the obit. Ordered the pinwheel sandwiches for after the service.

My dad, furious and ashamed at spending half his life dying, only to outlive his only son, stopped PKJ mid-stride and asked with barely contained fury, "What is it with you?"

"Pardon me?"

"You don't seem ... I mean, you seem ... all right. Are you, are you ... *over* this?"

Actual Me took this one. "What it is with me, is that I want my brother back. I want to make him not dead. I can't do that. So I am doing what I can."

He walked away.

More papers needed signing. PKJ offered to ride out to the funeral home with our "grief coordinator." As they cruised the highway around town, headed to the wide open spaces where crematoriums lived, actual Kelley stared at the rows of power pylons, holding up their skirts of humming lines. I spoke, startling everyone in the car.

"I know my mother said we weren't to look at the body. But I want to see him when we get there."

The grief coordinator even smelled scared.

"Um. He's not ... your parents consented to donate his eyes ... we didn't prepare him for viewing." And while you're freaking me out, you're not signing the cheques for this, was the silent finish, delivered with a turned head and a tightened grip on the steering wheel.

But my baby brother is cold. I want to wrap around him. Give him the heat of my body. Trust that it will bring him back to life. I won't care about the missing eyes, the broken sockets. He is little and alone, and there is nothing I will see that is worse than knowing that and not being able to do *something*.

I went back to watching the passing towers.

Sister Jess created an installation of Steve's artifacts for the funeral: cigarette lighters and stuffed toys and skull earrings and his guitar. Hundreds of packets of Dubble Bubble for the guests. His friends gave speeches loving and odd and simply confused, so confused to be in that crowded room, acting as if Steve was dead, because that was ridiculous. There was an awesome playlist. Eric emceed with grace. And during the invitation-to-speak section, my beautiful angry eldest son stood up, wearing his uncle's vest, without prep or warning.

"My uncle was cool. He gave me rides on his motorcycle. He would talk to me about stuff. He told me that the world was messed up, but there was a simple solution. Kill all the stupid people." That there was a huge laugh as a 13-year-old child recommended human culling tells you a bit about Steve, his friends, and how we raise kids in my family.

My mom, wild with the loss of the person that she loved the most in the world, threw me out of her house the night before. So I stood away from my parents as guests arrived and departed.

"Excuse me, can you tell me where the washrooms are?"

PKJ pointed to the left, happy to be mistaken for funeral home staff.

Riding to the motel we'd booked after Mom snapped, Actual Me crept into the quiet of the car interior, pressed my gloves to my face. Looked at Eric's face, lit by the dashboard. So real. So like himself. This *all* might be real. It might actually be happening.

Then I heard a crunch, like the sound the tube inside a glow stick makes breaking and releasing the light. I thought, dully, oh, it's my heart. That's a bit on the nose.

Home again. House things. Kid things. Saying things. Work. And then finally, alone. Silence.

"NO."

I paced my room and screamed that one word. Out loud. For 40 minutes.

Pam and I cart the inappropriately pink flowers to the Catholic side of the cemetery in Concord, New Hampshire, which is pretty much attached to Penacook, New Hampshire. Pam hurt her back fussing with her own gardens, getting ready for us to visit, so I am on the ground doing a terrible job of planting the flowers on my grandmother and grandfather's graves. The geraniums seem too small, and I'm crowding them, and I ask Pam anxiously if they're in right, and she does an "Oh, Kelley, whatever you want. It's fine." There are whiffs of Cotillion in the air as she sighs this out.

Then we go around to the other family graves, Uncle Jeff, my great uncles, and some cousins. See that others have already done us better on this Memorial Day weekend. Bigger flowers. Straightened American flags for the veterans.

I am rarely in graveyards these days. My mother has Steve's ashes. Dad was scattered over a frozen creek. Teen ... well, I am undecided about where Teen is. My dead are untendable.

I loved graveyards when I was little. It was one of the trips Teen and I would make most weeks, to one of the two Westminster graveyards that at one point my family owned. I loved stretching out under a small and terrifically twisted old hawthorn that hung over my ancestors, eyes half-closed to sun sieved through its branches. Teen fluttered, worried that somehow a 3-year-old on a grave was asking for trouble. But I would not be moved. There was power in the quiet earth, like the power I felt by the sea. So I laid my back into it, drew it up and into my spine.

I feel no inclination to do that here, in the Concord cemetery.

Why not? Crowded, inelegant, the Catholic side pushing up against the Prods', this graveyard is unlike the one in Westminster, but I have relatives everywhere. It's like a Burke family party here, all the aunts and uncles and cousins by the dozens ringing the place, insisting, one after another, on planting kisses that smell of cigarettes and Four Roses bourbon on my cheek. Hearty, loud townies — jolly with each other — seemingly simple and anything but. All together here, where the party ends. And I feel like I'm crashing it.

They always had each other. They've had so much of each other.

I look once more around the sunny graveyard, pour the last bit from a communal watering can on my Burke grandmother's inadequate flowers. I can do that much for her. (That much being nothing.) Shift in the steamy New England heat. Watch my aunt limp a bit as she heads back to her car. My aunt who did everything.

We delay leaving the next morning, so I can quickly grip my second cousin, Teddy, my Dad's age and one of his closest boyhood friends, who has rushed over to Pam's house to see me.

"You look like your fatha'," he says.

"You hug like him," I answer next to his ear as we hold each other hard and then let go hard, like something has begun to burn.

I am under-slept and teary and Teddy is clearly seeing dead people as he looks at me. I start to get dizzy. This old man (who will die within the year) has pulled his already hurting body into my aunt's dining room to see me. He offered me this love. This courtesy. And I am fainting, to leave. I have not felt this strong a need to do anything since ...?

Since I asked to see my brother's body a decade plus ago, the blood slamming in my temples answers.

I shake that nonsense off. The Nubble. The deal that was sealed when I was less than two. That's what I am rushing to. I simply need to get home-ish. Find my safe place. Fix whatever the hell I have that is broken. I get my bag rolling down the pathway into the rental car. My feet chatter on the floor mats and I wave like a regular person whose heart isn't threatening to jump out of her throat and run ahead of the vehicle.

That a nostalgia that provokes cardiac episodes may not be entirely healthy does *not* occur to me. And if it did, it is quickly dismissed.

Lunch, Interrupted 1996

Next morning, back at the cottage with my grandfather, having returned the pilfered papers, I am in Teen's closet, looking for photos. Eric has charged me with finding what I can of a family history that I have largely constructed rather than documented. The old man comes into her room for the first time since I've been here. I've noticed he doesn't even look towards her bedroom door when he walks past it to the john, proving that the murderer always returning to the scene of the crime is not a reliable maxim.

He watches me for a moment and then says, "You didn't have to come ... it was good a' you."

I freeze. I cannot think what to say. I see he has shaved, and know by the shine of his face that he is using the bone-handled straight razor yet. I smell his splash of witch hazel as aftershave. And then I am three and being lifted up past his brown plaid work shirt and against that leather cheek. Loving the clean wet wood tonic smell, the smoothness of his skin so different from my father's boyish stubble face. Loving him. My small arms fit nicely around the red, scraped neck. His oddly dainty ears, wrapped in the gold arms of his spectacles, pressing against my cheek. Oh, the old man was old when I was three, and now I'm thirty-four.

"You're my family, Grampa. Of course, I came. "

"Your grandmother ... she liked it when you came that other time."

"Yes, I know."

"I wish she hadn't of died."

"Me too."

"It's no good now."

"I miss Teen too."

And then he asks me to lunch.

I get ready in Teen's room. The clothes I'm wearing are for cleaning, not lunching, and nothing from Teen's collection of stretch suits and cruise wear is going to be much help. In the last years, she got broad in the belly—which was confusing because she was my thin grandmother, to the point where in earlier pictures you can see that it went from natural health to something else, something knife-edged and ruthless.

But after Teen went fully crazy and her constant fear left, she could eat. And the starved system seemed to hoard what it was given, lest she change her mind.

I go across to the old man's room, steal a clean white shirt and a belt and take them back to the smaller bedroom, throw them, with a bit of a wince, on Teen's bed. Not that it hasn't been cleaned since the death. Even the lacklustre cleaner could figure that one out. But because the crazy part of me suspects she's still lying there.

At the very back of her closet, I find a peasant skirt with an elastic waist, Mexican I think, blue with over-sized, over-bright thread flowers at the hem. A gift perhaps from a travelling friend who did not know my grandmother at all.

The skirt fits and goes with the shirt and belt. I open Teen's top drawer. I know exactly where to find the earrings. Next to the carnelians, in the box with the Victorian hair brooches that she never wore but were "good" and so important: a set of rhinestone clip-ons, pink pineapple-shaped sprays. They are the sparkly remnants of a great gal, a once-upon-a-time free spirit, who would get on the train and ride from Westminster to Harlem to shimmy in the clubs. Play the banjo and busk for change with her best friend. Dress in fire engine red sequined splendor, glittering bandeaux over forehead and at the ears, like exquisite ear muffs. I clip on their glittery splendor. Then I stop. I'm stealing. I'm stealing my dead grandmother's stuff.

The old man won't let me have anything of Teen's; I've asked. It's not like I want anything valuable. Something familiar, I tell him. A mumbled "No," and stomping off...leaving me cod-mouthed. Now I set my lips and quietly tell myself that this is not theft but salvage.

I pull my hair in a ponytail, reach, without thought, for hairpins that are surely in the wooden box on her bureau top. And come out of the room looking, I have to say, quite smart. My grandfather stares and for a lurching moment, I think he's noticed the stolen swag on my ears. But then he says:

"You look like your mother."

"Thanks Grampa."

He nods, seems to find his bolo tie too tight and is busy adjusting it for a moment, and then stomps over to the door. The phone rings. Speaking of Mom.

"Is he dead yet?" she asks.[23]

"No. We're on our way to lunch."

"Oh. That's nice."

"The neighbours think maybe he's having little strokes. He's fallen a few times."

Silence. As he goes through the door, I register something in my grandfather's hand. To Mom. "He needs someone to come in. He shouldn't be alone in the house at all."

"Find anything good?"

"Define good."

"Is the jewellery still there? The good stuff?"

I touch the rhinestone confections already making my lobes ache. And then hear my rental car rev.

"Oh god, Mom, he's got my car keys. I've got to go."

---

23. See entire next chapter.

"Is he dead yet?" — An Extremely Long Footnote on the Subject of Memory (with a horse) 2018

YOU: (looking up from the manuscript) "She said what?"

ME: "Is he dead yet ..."

YOU: "And ..."

ME: "If I'd found anything good."

YOU: "Who are you people?????"

Okay. Fair question—to be clear, I'm not sure that my mother said that. I've told the story of this trip more than a few times, and I remember her leading with "Is he dead yet?" but I cannot swear

I didn't make that one up. It sure *sounds* like a conversation we would have. It sounds like who *we* were. But memory is a bitch.

For example, before Eric and I leave Penacook, I remind Pam about a story she told me, years earlier, about my cousin Sarah. In first or second grade, she wrote something for class about her sister Cathy's pets (many pets) and the way the Burke Family compound adapted to life as an animal refuge. About the bunny room on the second floor, stacked Rapunzel-high with cast-off mattresses in which a 20 lb rabbit dug and burrowed. About the endless lizards and dogs and tamed feral cats. About the horse who moved from the old barn to the under-repair and wall-knocked-out spare kitchen —

"That didn't happen."

"What?"

"Didn't happen."

"Sarah wrote the story about your house and her teacher sent a note home saying what a wonderful imagination Sarah had. And you sent a note back saying: "No. She doesn't.""

"Yes. I did that. And we had the rabbit upstairs. And all those other pets. And there was a horse. But it stayed in the barn."

"I completely remember the horse in the kitchen —"

"Yes."

"Cathy was re-doing the gyprock in the spare kitchen —"

"Uh huh."

" — and the back wall was off, so the horse came in, for the winter."

"Sweetie, you write it any way you want. But it didn't happen."

"I guess you wouldn't have left the back off the house in the winter ..."

"Or left a horse in my kitchen."

See, I thought she would. My aunt and uncle were so amazingly accepting in a John Irving-esque "we're all a little bit from the circus and we don't play by the rules" sort of way that that's exactly what I thought they would do. And I loved them for it. But wasn't the bunny room enough? An entire room for a pet rabbit? Scuffing up mattress guts as it dug yet another tunnel, excreting a full expression of a rabbit life into the two hundred year old floorboards? You'd think I wouldn't feel the need to tart that one up. But evidently I did. My wonderful, mad family in New England, whom I loved and who loved me—you can see the children's book cover, can't you? I think the horse has a unicycle.

I read an article by a professor named Giuliana Mazzoni of the University of Hull that broke down her findings from a large and robust study of how humans use their memory. She says that memory is not a filing cabinet—it is an art exhibit, carefully curated by the psyche—with pieces chosen (or culled or amended) to support the current iteration of who we *believe* we are.

There are people with super-memories who can play back almost anything if you give them the code they file under, like dates. Walk up to one of them and say June 12, 2003, 9AM—and they will tell you that they ate cereal and an orange for breakfast, and that they are at that time in the bathroom at work, mopping a spill off their blouse, acquired as they drove over a pothole while sipping a cup of Timmy's (which, I would explain to my American cousins, is the Canadian Dunkin's) with a loose lid. But that is an incredibly rare ability—and once the party trick has run its course, a dull one. No radiant light of universal understanding there. No hilarious insight. It's security camera footage. Who wants total recall of every time they sat on the toilet? Picked their nose and tried to find a place to hide the results? Considered getting up and starting breakfast and thought, why me? instead kicking their partner and faking sleep, mouth slightly agape, before said partner figured out why they were awake.[24]

We instead tend to hold onto that which we feel best illustrates the story of ourselves. And that changes over time—both in what we choose to hold and the integrity of what we hold.

Some stuff is more insistent on being retained intact. Firsts.

---

24. I know. That example is over-specific. Move along.

Onlys. Actual scars. So ... first recess, grade one playground—my sweaty little chub hands reaching and losing the metal dividing bar of the whirling merry-go-round. Looking at a boy sitting at the centre of the spinning wheel. "Help me," I plead. The relief at his smile. The blood as he kicks me in the face, and I still hold on, and am dragged, bare-kneed, over gravel. A memory permanently inscribed into my nose. My knees. A memory of cruelty. Before the memory-go-round (I was trying to write merry-go-round, but I like that better), cruel did not exist for me. Not for real. Cruel was Cinderella's step-mother, and Mr. McGregor and his pies, and Boris and Natasha, drawn in crayon colours on TV screens, but not in the world. And then it was. So I remember this. And whenever I go through a similar conjunction of pain, humiliation and flat out disbelief at cruelty, the memory freshens, moves back up to the top of the retention queue, because it is both physically concrete and *chosen* as the illustration of a particular chapter in what I believe, at a deep and usually unexamined level, is the Story of Me.

But with other memories, as self-perception changes, so do the recollections. Things that remained forgotten when I thought I was someone else, I begin to remember when they confirm who I think I am now. Just not necessarily as they happened. Ergo, I wanted a life in which there was a horse in the kitchen. So I remembered one.

There is no intention to re-construct reality. It just happens. And it gets more complicated. Because even as I have collected and curated my memories of the Story of Me, so have those around me—as they wrote their own draft of themselves, and me. To the point where the whole business of me is more debate than definition. E.G.:

The Story of Kelley, Stephen's Sister, age ten:

KELLEY: *I wake up to the second or third scream. The sharpened hook is in Steve's throat, cannibal teeth tear at the wound and he screams again, caught in the nightmare he has every night for three hot summer weeks.*

This began with a YMCA summer weekend sleepaway. First night, a couple of counsellors tell the tale of the Camp Manitou Tramp before lights out in the teepee. They describe the hook, the oven where the deranged hobo roasts his captured children, the mothers weeping over the bones found in the ashes. Then they take all the flashlights and leave, waiting an hour or so before drag-limping slowly around the outside of the tent, raking a "claw" over the fabric, then slowly raising the zipper using the end of what was a straightened coat hanger. Eight pissed-in sleeping bags and two kids sent home at midnight because they couldn't stop barfing later and the counsellors saw the error of their ways.

Our family was still seeing it with Steve, around 2AM every night. Soaking the bed. Screaming for help. All without being truly awake.

I could hear my father starting his sleep-cursing. "GEEEE-Sus. KEErist! Gawd DAAAM!" He's not awake either but Dad asleep and angry is way worse. He will thunder and pound the door frame and Steve will cry harder. I have to get there first.

I slip out of bed. Into Steve's room. He's still light enough for me to carry. I pull him into in a rock-a-bye baby hold, half-awake, his face wet and swollen. Stagger down the hall. Make sure not to trip over his Boo Bankie (blue blanket, essential and irreplaceable). Kind of loving the way his nose looks for the crook of my neck.

Lay him at the foot of my bed, quivering, not quite sure where he is, and moving into the shuddering calm after the sob. Wrap him in the Boo.

"Okay. Go to sleep now. I'm right here." And move back into my own sleep, feet tucked to give him room ...

The Story of Kelley, Stephen's Sister, age ten:

STEVE: *No. No more. Her knees on my shoulders. Her fingers in my ribs, under my arms. Scream. Scream. I am laughing but I am not laughing. I can't bear it. I can't. Louder, higher. Anything to get Mom to come in and stop her. I can't get her off me. She smells of girl sweat and ginger snaps — and she is laughing, her face hanging over me, hectic and blotchy. And she is so heavy.*

And she loves this. Look at her. Swelling up like a tick with everything she's taking from me. I hate her. I hate her. I hate how I scream when she even moves her finger like she is going to tickle me. A yard away from me.

That's all it takes. She wiggles her finger and I laugh shriek run.

But I don't run this time. Don't squeal like her little pig. This time
I hit, in the belly, hard, and then she slams me down.

If I don't get away I will die.

Bite.

She slaps, hard on the mouth, like I'm a dog. She's bleeding. Good.
Run now, with loud loud crying. Mom will kill her, because she hit
my face. Maybe I'll have a bruise. That would be better. Anything would
be better.

I will kill her someday. For now—the blood on my teeth will do,

Both those stories happened. Both are factually true and can be
confirmed by witnesses. The person in the 1st story and the person
in the 2nd story seem to have little to do with each other. Protector.
Torturer. Safety from the night storm. Tick. After years of raising
my own children, I will generally offer the first story as an illustration of who I was as a child. Steve did offer the 2nd, regularly, when
he was alive, and made himself available to my kids as the advisor
he knew they would need in their life with their (inevitably) abusive
mother.

Each story is mostly fiction as well. Emotional flashes and torn
pictures that we push and twist together until they look as we
thought they ought. And of course, Steve's version is filtered through
my memory of how he described me to me, to my kids ... so doubly
constructed and selected and curated and groomed ...

Dr. Mazzoni says to go with the constructs of memory that make
you happy. Go with your best version of how you remember yourself.
Try to be that self. Hang out with people willing to remember you
that way. Embrace the curation.

Sounds like great advice—for a Nazi hanging out in an Argentinian
cantina hoping no one notices his accent. Or a homesick kid who
wants to tell you about the horse in the kitchen.

The Addams 2020

So who were we people (before Dad got sick, because, after that, we were something else)?

Well, we were ... odd. Off. Immune, by design, to the community norms that bind "nice" people. When we moved to Canada, we could have been the Burkes Who Walked Out. The Abandoners. The Deadbeat Bukes. My family chose something other. Not the combined family burdens of guilt and class and what families hold due. Not Burkes. Not Adams. But Addams:

(Wait for it. Get your fingers ready...)

Snap. Snap.

They're creepy and they're kooky
Mysterious and spooky
They're all together ooky
The Addams family.

It's on. Everything stops. This is the best show *ever*. This makes being in Canada bearable. This is about us. Let's do it together.

Their house is a museum
When people come to see them
They really are a scream
The Addams family

(and the Addams on the screen hold perfectly still, stare straight into the camera, not so much menacingly as sublimely *other*-ly, hands in position, fingers poised to ...)

 Snap. Snap.

If you missed the original series, or more likely weren't alive when it aired (1964-65, though it lived on in re-runs for many years) and only have access to the inferior films and Nickelodeon reboots, *The Addams Family* was an absurdist sitcom about a dark, deliciously happy family with, to me, perfectly logical interests: moon bathing, feeding the carnivorous plants, owning a pet lion named "Kitty Cat," giving racks and guillotines test runs (they don't make 'em like the used to) and duelling as foreplay. They had a servant named Lurch who was seven feet tall, a hell of an organist, and quite possibly a re-animated corpse, a cousin was a gibbering haystack of hair, and another, an amputated hand that mixed a mean cocktail.

It was so nice to spend time with people like us.

Channel 12 in Winnipeg carried all kinds of odd bits of syndi-cation, and, one day, a year or two after we moved to Canada, the original Addams Family, much loved when we were still in the u.s., showed up there. And we all stood around the TV and warmed our hands by the black and white moonlight and snap snapped our fin-gers along with our *kin*. Celebrated and codified and swore alle-giance to chosen eccentricity. We continued to go by Burke. But in disposition and displacement we were something else. We were the Addams Family North.

Any time one of us opened our mouths in small town, rough cut late 60s Winnipeg, we proclaimed our Addams-ness, not by our lan-guage or food or music (though our household, made up of objects that Canadians called antiques and we called furniture, was a clear clue that we were *not from these parts*. Of course we weren't. Parts were for other people) but by our indifference to what was and was not *done*. We scorned people who were guided by anything other than the logic and self-interest that led us to emigrate. You know. Family. Decency. Faith. What the neighbours would think. All that malarkey.

My university counsellor dad was the steady one in our Addams cast. He had a straight job, left in the morning and came home at night like the other dads, sipping the lowball Johnny Walker I knew to bring in a round, heavy-bottomed glass, one ice cube and a trickle of water. But he didn't wear short sleeve shirts and tie clips and or carry a briefcase. He ran group encounter sessions in the Manitoba bush, sported a dashiki, puka beads and a man-of-the-mountains beard. Occasionally he would come home from one "encounter" or another needing medical attention:

"Tell me again why you need this injection, James?'

"One of the participants —"

"A girl."

"Yes, a girl. She has Hep B, and so everyone who —"

"Bodily fluid. You need to have been in contact with bodily fluid."

"She was crying Ruth!"

"Yes?"

"For like ... four hours."

"Uh huh."

"In my lap."

"Ah."

My mother cultivated her own brand of proto-feminism—which included no interest at all in being equal with men, as she had no wish to lower herself, a not entirely metaphorical belief in her own capacity for witchcraft, and raising hell and saying *anything* in the suburbs. She got investigated for hitting a kid, full force, who was beating on the post-surgery stitches of another boy's eye. She told the bully to stop. He gave her the finger. She knocked him into Tuesday. The bully's mom told the cops everyone knew my mom was a nut job. The bully's father, who worked for Eye Stitches' dad, told his wife to shut up. Mom sewed a long black gown like Morticia Addams' to wear for Halloween, and laid in some dry ice for the bowl of holiday punch.

We children were a mix of the two—counter-culture, violent, and arcane. Steve was a biting, giggling, anarchic little weasel, haunted by demons. I was a chubby goody two shoes with a bent for showing off and throwing down, but only in the service of righteousness. Jess, the youngest, was our Lurch, silent, head-shaking and ultimately the master of secretive acts of revenge (my favourite involved punishing my pilfering brother by filling his bed with something? cereal and milk? wet leaves? when she knew he would be coming home drunk). We competed viciously for our mother's love and often hated each other (Steve's early acquisition of a book on psychological warfare was of great use to him in and out of the home). He schemed, I slugged, and Jess bided her time and knew that vengeance was a dish best served cold. And damp.

But that was between us. The rest of the world was another matter. Torment my brother and you'd be on your ass, heat-butted by me, or clothes-lined by Jess. Look at my sister wrong, and Steve would smile and say "I will end you." (And mean it. After one of his friends was jumped and beaten senseless, my brother had a chat with the local psychopath and the beater's knee caps were shattered. This was reported to Jess and I, and each of us just nodded. Yup. That's how that should go.) And when a young heller on our street called my person-of-colour sister a word that started with N and threw dog shit at her, I broke his collarbone.

We lived in the shadows, spoke like renaissance gentlemen, and would have worked well in black and white.

So put a witch's shawl on
A broomstick you can crawl on
We're going pay a call on
The Addams family

Odd. That's how I remember us. Deliberately, consciously odd. And it required each and every one of us to put away any not-odd feelings about the inconvenient truths and inconvenient people we'd left behind, so that we might write a new and whimsical story of ourselves.

And so we *knew* the Burkes could look after themselves, and Teen was a silly drunk who'd made her Grampa-bed and should lie in it, and none of them *really* liked us, and it was well we were away.

To do know anything else was bad and disloyal. And could result in all manner of familial retribution.

And I gave in to that bit of curation, for the right to be let in, and snap along with the rest of the cast. I put all the longing for that which we were supposed to leave behind, into the one receptacle I could not relinquish, addict that I was. I put it all into the lighthouse. And that was permitted me, as it was also fairly and safely odd.

Snap. Snap.

The Rat 2018

"I couldn't sleep and I was afraid of waking you."

We are in the rental car, flying towards Cape Neddick, having left Penacook later than planned.

We've been two days in a house that didn't really have room for us, as one of Pam's guest rooms is in use (her grandkids' vast collection of Lego is permanently resident, leaving the room a nubbed plastic block minefield). But rather than say no, and send us to a motel, Pam settled two largish adults in her one remaining, smallish guest bed. By the second night, overlapping painfully, inland New England heat wave heavy on our skin—sleep was impossible. After the third time waking up with Eric's forearm smashed into my bazoo (he flails in his sleep), I started to freak.

"So I went to the Lego room."

I'm telling Eric the story of the night before because despite his ability to walk, talk, and on more than one occasion, fulfill his conjugal duties mid-REM, Eric rarely remembers the things that happen in the night. This boggles me. I go from sleep to complete wakefulness in less than a second and have perfect recall of all dark time adventures, most of them anxiety-fuelled and embarrassing. And, as such, something that must be kept quiet until daylight chases the shame off. Then it is equally imperative that I put them out in the world, because until Eric knows where I was while he slept, some part of me is still there.

And so this extended storytelling as we leave New Hampshire and head out to York Beach:

I pick my way through the Lego, lie down and try to sleep. The windows are still stretch-sealed from the winter, and it is dusty and stuffy. Cough. Never mind.

Scritch. A scrabbling in the walls. Racoon? I wonder. Scratch. Rat, I decide. I will ignore it, because I am probably crazy and there is no rat. Scritch, scratch, scuffle. It will crawl on me if I sleep. It will eat my face like that guy in 1984. Scratch. Jump up and stand, wrapped in soft dusty heat, with no idea what to do next.

I go back to our room. Start looking for my shoes, cell phone. I will try downstairs. Sleep on a couch.

But one of the things about beautiful, relatively untouched New England 19th century homes like my aunt's is the back staircases are ... special. Time-smoothed wooden triangles the size of moderate slices of pizza, wedged into a tiny helix stack; they were for the servants, who apparently were expected to have very small feet. They are impossible to walk in the dark, and the stairwell light is burned out. The hand railing is also broken, because Pam lives in a heritage site, and there are always more repairs needed than time. With my arthritis-numbed feet and hands, I will surely die, in the dark, on the stairs.

I don't want to wake you, obviously, because I am a smart person. I know better than to inflict sleep-robbing crazy on tomorrow's designated driver. So I am fumbling for my shoes. Quietly. Fairly quietly. Sniveling. Also what some would describe as quietly. Wondering when the hell you're going to wake up.

Sob.

Nothing.

Long drawn out shudder.

Nothing.

Oops. I drop my shoe.

Bingo. You wake up.

I tell you about the Lego room, how it was hot and the dust was choking me. And the rat. Especially the rat.

You doubt the rat immediately.

I agree. Obviously there is no rat. I am totally making up the rat. But I am going downstairs because I can't sleep with the rat. Except I am afraid that I will die on the way down. I didn't want to wake you. I am not that selfish, except I clearly am because I know you're going to offer to go downstairs instead of me, because that's the sort of thing you do, and that makes me feel instantly calmer, which is why I've woken you. And I am not smart and was never pretty. And soon you will not like me at all any more.

Next Day Eric, listening to the story as he drives, rolls his eyes. And then calmly avoids three potential pile-ups in as many moments. I look at him.

"So of course you do it. You say you *like* the couch."

He grins.

No, I think. It's not fair. You need the sleep more than me. I should be brave and responsible and adult and do the sensible thing here.

"Okay." Snivel.

Middle-of-the-night You gather up your apnea stuff. I grab my cell phone (the light app at the ready) and follow because at the very least I will light my beloved's way. Make sure you can see as you go down the death stairs. But you don't go to the death stairs, you go to THE RAT ROOM! No! I think. But you're in and on the bed.

I'm ashamed. Head back to the now comfy guest room, and lie by the window, cool and dust free and all I can think is: you won't be able to sleep. And when we drive the Number 4 tomorrow in Memorial weekend grid, you will try so hard, but it will only be a second's loss of consciousness — I have seen you do this — you will drop asleep at the wheel, still hand-clenched and foot on the gas, and we will die in a fiery blaze and leave our children trying to get our crispy, mangled bodies across the border. Jessie, the eldest, will try to be efficient and Sam, the middle, will be angry and Finn, our youngest, who is on the autism spectrum, will look around trying to figure out how he is supposed to react because he's learned that neurotypicals have very specific protocols for this sort of thing and his impulses are not his friends.

And it will hurt.

I sit rigid and poised for liftoff in the dark. Clench the phone in case you change your mind and try the stairs. Or in case you think better of it and come back down the hall, because you could trip and fall trying to find the guest room, as you stumble, exhausted and angry and ready to punt me out the window.

I am dripping sweat and the adrenaline headache is kicking in. I hear a couple of little coughs from down the hall, and that makes stars burst behind my eyes—the dust is making you ill. We are so gonna die tomorrow.

Next Day Eric gets us off I93, and onto #4 which is really just a winding two-lane horse and buggy road connecting dozens of inland New Hampshire towns with Portsmouth and the sea without incident.

After a half an hour I hear you snore. At least you're sleeping. It won't be good sleep and the apnea will make you a vegetable and I will be a brain widow but we've dodged the fiery car crash. And I am so greedy. Weak. Rats in my belfry.

Eric is not an actual saint[25], and it's not always this bad. I am usually able to manage my anxiety without daily medication—which is good, because I have never found one without unacceptable side effects. I practice breath management, visualization, physical relaxations, things I now teach (those who can, do, those who can't, offer sessional courses). Get regular exercise ... regular sleep ... and

---

25. Like the proverbial duck, he simply has a rare and beautiful capacity to let my verbal tsunamis crash and run off his mental back.

short-term medication that works when I need it. Most of the time, it's okay.

But travel makes it worse, and leading up to this trip, I was in a state of what I call "pop n' fresh" sleeplessness. Dropping off, and then "popping" awake moments later, heart a' thunder, over and over, with my own voice screaming at me—something like this:

WAKE UP!!!

    WHAT?

    HOW CAN YOU SLEEP?

    Sweat sweat.

    Pay attention.

    Youaresofuckedup

    But what but if but then but what but if...

    WHY ARE YOU SLEEPING WHEN YOU SHOULD BE SOLVING?!

    Toss

    IS THE CAT IN THE OVEN?

    What is the BEEPING?

    I will never I can never it will never...

    "WHATIF!!!!!!

    Are you crazy?

    You are better than... this calm down... draw it in and out... see the facts and ...and ... and ... breathe ...

    WAKE UP?!!!

    WHAT? HOW CAN YOU SLEEP? Sweat sweat Pay attention Youaresofuckedup But what but if but then but what but if... WHYAREYOUSLEEPINGWHENYOUSHOULDBESOLVING?!

    Toss

    IS THE CAT IN THE WASHER? What is the BEEPING? I will never I can never it will never... WHATIF!!!!! Are you crazy? You are better than this calm down... draw it in and out... see the facts and ... and ... and ... breathe ...

    WAKE UP?!!!"

Rinse. Repeat.

And so I was not ... at my best.

Since being afraid of an actual thing is *great* compared to the omnipresent smothering and too huge-to-be-known generalised anxiety that renders me sleepless, I was putting a lot of time into identifying things that I could rightfully dread and give my exponentially amping panic a name and shape and right of egress. Fear of flying. Fear of being seized at the border and put in a cage. Fear of Gabrielle the owner awaiting us on the steps of the cottage, yelling "Psych!", yanking the keys away, and chasing us off the property.

What I needed was to break up with my brain. To go into a coma. At least lose consciousness. A couple of weeks before we left, I asked Eric if he would have sex with me so hard that he knocked me out. You know, do a sister a solid. I may have asked more than once. Perhaps happily, he found the request off-putting.

The Teen tradition would have been to drink and pill myself into a stupor, but I could not be doing that. I had a kid still living at home, this husband who deserved better, and a deep belief that a middle-aged blowsy drunk will at some point morph into Liz Taylor in *Who's Afraid of Virginia Woolf?* and nobody wants that.

As a child, I thought we were all like this. I thought spending days and nights visualizing catastrophe and fighting for air was the human condition. Then I found out that any number of you, if anything, don't spend nearly *enough* time anticipating the potentially tragic consequences of mundane actions. [26]

Why am I like this? Why am I "just like Teen?"

One theory. I was born this way.

A study conducted at the Worcester Polytechnic Institute (which is a half hour drive from where I was born) showed evidence that experiences like childhood abuse, deprivation, and traumatic fear can make changes at the DNA level of someone's makeup, becoming part of the epigenetic package that is handed to following generations.

---

26. This sentence brought to you by the year 2020.

The research was done by shocking sea slugs to see if their grand-children were born nervous. Spoiler: they were. So, the theory extends, my grandmother Teen's crushing anxiety may be ribonucleic acid-etched on my psyche.

It must be said first that most of the shocks that I know about that could have affected Teen's slug happened *after* my mom was born. Mom was her only child to survive after multiple miscarriages, and, in early life, was sickly to the point of sadism. Allergic to everything—wool, grass, mold, milk—they bought Mom a goat or she would have starved as an infant. As she nursed Mom through tonsillitis (Mom was also allergic to penicillin as it turns out), measles, a broken arm, a ruptured appendix, Teen became a clutching, twisting, terrified mess with a sometimes discreet pill and booze addiction and a frequent flyer card at the dipsomania sanatorium. My mother rejected any suggestion of frailness and was a climber of trees, shooter of guns, a rider of Horses of Death (all horses were Horses of Death, according to Teen). I'm not saying Mom lay in bed as a child, thinking of ways to send Teen into the looney bin; I'm just saying, if you look at pictures of my mother as a girl, hair a Shirley temple mop, a Rockwell picture of innocence, remember, the Devil comes in pleasing forms.

But those shocks are moot as far as *my* genetic inheritance goes. I think there must have been shocks that came before. Teen was born timid and tiny, to parents who were of the hard-work-and-lots-of-whipping school of child-rearing. She had a couple of near death experiences as a child that I know about—trampling by a Horse of Death, almost-drownings, falls. Her mother had a pretty horrible and soul-slamming life as well, including a cross-the-sea voyage from England as a replacement bride for the man her sister had died trying to reach on an earlier crossing. So I think it is completely possible Teen's sea slug was shocked unto the seventh generation. I think I come from a long line of flinching gastropods, and that Teen's sizzling genes passed intact to me. I think my first-born thought, as I slug-slithered out of the womb, was "ZAP!" immediately followed by "AAAAAAAH!"

Or, and this is theory two, Teen *made* me like this.

Teen was my primary person, early on. My mother kept me clean and fed and beautifully dressed and taught me as she was taught. But Mom was probably depressed after that horrible birth, and living next door to difficult parents who hated her new husband, and whose family hated her. If I'd been in that situation, I'd have screamed all day. Rolled in bees. Or done exactly what my mother did, fight for some semblance of her old independence, and once she was pregnant again, and vilely sick (pregnancy was no more a picnic for Mom than labour), frickin' sleep on the brown couch in the dappled afternoon sun, as much as possible, and let baby me toddle off to Teen.

She was right next door, running her insurance business (because what the clinically anxious *need* is regular exposure to actuarial tables showing the odds on all the ways people can die). I could hang out there, or head over to great-grandmother Jessie, in the house on the other side of mine, her butter mints in a pewter dish and a box of fabulous spiny sea shells from Florida on her back kitchen porch to keep me busy. Or there was my great-grandfather sitting in his "summer house", a collapsible screened-in one season structure where he went to drink a little apple jack, smoke a pipe, and dodge the more challenging family dynamics.

But mostly there was Teen, reaching, "Little hand in big hand, Kelley!" taking me for the daily walk down to Main Street, into Johnny's Market, and then to the library, and, on Sundays, the First Congregational Church. I think when little hand was in big hand she didn't worry about me getting killed. I think it may have been the only time.

There were so many lightning rods spiking our roofs when I was little that no one else in Westminster got so much as a glance from the storm god. He knew a welcome mat when he saw one. If it wasn't the lightning that needed to be anticipated, then it was the spaces in her attic where there was no floor, only exposed rafters and the wires and lathe of the kitchen ceiling ("You'll fall right through, honey, and get hurt so bad"). If not that, there was the barn swing, the flagstone wall, all foot and a half of it, or especially the old well, no longer used now that we were on the town water system. It was capped by a gigantic grind stone that once spun to sharpen tools, but now simply covered the hole.

I loved lying on that huge stone wheel on sunny days—it was baking warm and the constant ants a never-ending engagement. If I was very still, I could hear the gurgle and clop of the water, far below, catch breaths of cold wet seeping up between the stone and the earth. The idea of lying suspended above a secret sea was irresistible. The grind stone weighed hundreds of pounds, but Teen knew I would find a way to move it, and plummet down to a dark watery death. She could see it. So clearly.

"Kelley, you stay off that. Take my hand. Here. You are too precious."

Fantastic. Tears fell from Teen's squeezed-in-terror eyes as I was grabbed. Hugged. Snatched from the jaws of death. What drama. What significance. What can I be snatched from next? Death was all around, waiting. Teen said so. And it was thrilling.

Nature? Nurture? A predisposition fed by context? One well and truly shocked slug? However it happened, a hysteric was born.

I understand that being this way makes me less than admirable. I know what the right qualities for the heroine of any story are: kindness, generosity, rueful insight, bookish but undeniable good looks, and above all, courage. And I have none of those.

What I have is the one form of lying I still allow myself. I am a classic "high functioner." I fake brave and am stunned by how often people buy it. Am in constant fear of the moment when they catch me in the fake. The shame I will feel. Fearing that shame. Fearing that the fear of the shame will be what gets me caught faking ... which is another thing to fear ... oh never mind. You get the picture. Just this ridiculous scrabble up the nightmare clock face, again. Watching the waves' viscous horror spin below. Again.

Thinking this time I will just let go.

Back to the car, and telling Eric about the Rat.

I sat there after you left, basically waiting for whatever was going to eat me to make its move, because that's how I felt, like something was going to eat me. And don't say one rat couldn't eat me. Humans evolved able to produce these huge bursts of adrenaline that I get so we could run away from big prehistoric cats that loved to eat people better than anything. And sure there are no more big cats, but my heart doesn't know that. It's still ready. Pumped and slamming out of my chest like a rat in a meat cage. And if you make a cat/rat pun at this moment I will kill you.

Silence.

Nothing moved. No cats. No rats. That's when I decided I was making myself anxious over what was a non-issue. And it might be okay to take an Ativan.

Eric turns the steering wheel. "You think?"

"Uh huh. But the thing is, Eric, Teen was like that *all* the time."

I feel the car swing into the turn onto Old Market Road (the air cools and smells salt), and then on to Long Sands (hear the gulls, feel the waves before I see them), that will take us onto the coast road to her house. Eric reaches over and takes my hand. I look down at his, over mine.

When the Rat came for Teen ... there was no Eric. No hand. She was told to shut up and stop being so *stupid*. Like one ought with an invisible-rat-fearing, anxiety-zapped wreck. Of course she drank. Of course she took pills. With drink. She was looking for her coma. She was looking for a way to break up with her brain. Get the rat to shut up, for one blessed minute. And instead, she was mocked. And dismissed. And left behind — by me.

I don't tell Eric to drive faster. But as the lighthouse comes into view, I barely notice, occupied as I am with silently begging him to press on the gas.

The rat has her.

I have to get in.

Lunch, Continued (Honk) 1996

He revs the engine.

"Grampa. This is a rental car—I'm the only one who can drive it."

The old man lost his license after Teen died. Arthritic and with almost no discernable circulation to his feet, he'd been a questionable driver for years, unable to shoulder check, or temper his speed.

This combined with his basic choleric nature, poor eyesight, and, after Teen's death, blind terror led to the incident in Portsmouth, New Hampshire. He always went over the state line for groceries to evade Maine's higher taxes and tourist town prices. He parked right in front of the store and on leaving, mistook R for D, and gunned the car directly into and through a plate glass window, the stacks of Coal King briquettes, and the ice cooler, halting only at a checkout stand (and accompanying clerk).

At this point, Grampa *found* R. Gunned it. And fled the scene.

It took a fine paid, an apology offered, and a license revoked, for the family lawyer to keep him out of jail. But that didn't keep him off the road.

So the lawyer, a delightful, knowing man who seemed to get a kick out of Grampa, got into the habit of visiting Sundays. At some point, he'd slip down to the garage, and quietly pull something loose in the old man's engine. A rotor. A battery cable. A few spark plugs. Anything hard to see that would keep the car dead.

I shudder to think who Grampa blamed, probably at the top of his lungs, for the steady sabotage of his car. Summer people. Black people. Black summer people. Not his nice white lawyer certainly. He'd call 911, howl and tell the police to replace the part (this is how he lost his emergency call privileges—unofficially probably ...). When he got *someone* to help him, he would fix the car. But that took time, generally long enough for the lawyer to come round, and break something else.

So he became slowed the last year, if not completely immobilized.

But now, the old man is at the wheel of my fully functional rental, and is pulling out of his lane, honking.

"Hurry up." (honk)

"Grampa. I'm the only one who's allowed to drive this."

"Never mind about that." (honk)

"Grampa, I have to—" I open the passenger door to talk to him, his being locked, and he starts to back out. I am thrown into the seat, and grab at the door, which swings with the force of the old man gassing her out of the driveway.

HONK.

This is the oncoming car whose path he backs into, but he ignores this, gives the car a grinding shift, and heads down Nubble Road.

"*Oh Kelley, take care,*" Teen is not rumbling in my ear but squeaking (The whale thing has really not done the job, it seems. Maybe there's something else I have to do?). The old man favours straddling the yellow line, satisfied with half right at any given time. He's doing 50 miles an hour, which on the narrow winding cliff side route, bustling with early summer traffic, is heart-stopping. I wonder if seizing the wheel will save me, or get me killed faster.

"Let's go to Fox's." Fox's is in Sohier Park, the next left.

"It's no damn good. They charge you plenty and don't give you nuthin' you can't get for half the price."

"Grampa, you're really not supposed to drive my car. *Please* switch with me."

The old man shakes his head, taps his hearing aids.

"These don't work too good over the car. Tell me when we get there."

I speak louder but notice that he is speeding up every time I try to get him off the wheel. Teen is no longer talking to me, but I let out a series of clenched shrieks that I swear come straight from her. I edge my left foot towards the middle of the car floor so I can slam the brake, over his foot, if need be. Lock my shoulders for impact and watch the cliffs and sea and beach go by, trying to print it on my eyes. I hope the coroner will lift the picture from my lenses, print it up, show it to everyone.

Off the shoreline, and up Cape Neddick Road, winding up to the turnpike. We pass through a school zone. What time is it? I look at my watch—ten minutes until the school kids are out for lunch—please god let there have been no early dismissal. Then without shoulder checking, without even decreasing speed, he swings us onto the freeway.

We're using two out of three lanes, and cars are honking in fury—the speed limit's fifty-five, but no one is doing less than seventy. One more time:

"I want to drive," I'm starting to cry.

Up to eighty.

"— shut — I'm fine." The other cars are frightening the old man, so he is running away, his feet so numb that he probably can only guess at how much he is accelerating. Just going. Putting what terrifies him (and so must not be because he cannot be terrified, not in a right and orderly world) behind. Tears in his eyes as well. The underpasses have speed displays as you pass through. Eighty-five mph. The sign's alarm lights dance.

"Please slow —"

Eighty-seven. Where the hell is the highway patrol?

At the speed he's going it's less than fourteen minutes to Ogunquit and the exit. Clutching the dashboard, fourteen minutes is impossibly long. Hours. Days. I send a silent goodbye to Eric. My children. And then, "There's the turn-off!" I squeal.

I see the panic on the old man's face. *He doesn't know if he can brake.* Drags his foot off the gas. Slams over lanes. Car from behind swerving, drivers putting whole bodies onto car horns—one Neon full of terrified teenagers, perhaps out for their first try on the turnpike, follow the rental, shrieking and giving the old man the finger. No deceleration. None at all. I am paralyzed, watching us head for the trees beyond. Then his foot finds the brake and slams right down to the floor. I grab the wheel and crank it over. The old man doesn't even see me, has his eyes closed, pulling against my yank.

And then we are sitting, idling, about 20 yards down the turn-off. A restaurant is dead ahead.

"Well, there it is." And the old man hits the gas again and bangs the car over to the parking lot—straight over—two flower beds and a white decorative plastic chain are history. We stop with a thunk and a shudder somewhere around the middle, and he heaves himself out of the car, stumps towards the restaurant without a backwards glance.

The restaurant is windowless, WASP, and dark. Round backed frontier chairs. Brown plaid benches. Wagon wheels? Within spitting distance of a harbour? Welcome to the Good Ship Ponderosa. An elegant man in his forties greets us. Our waiter. He gives the sense that in the time it takes to gracefully walk us from the entrance to our table, he has sussed out the entire situation: my red cheeks, Grampa's set jaw, hammer fists hanging from his shoulders like meat clock pendulums. He hands us heavy leather-bound menus.

I don't need food. I need sedation. I order chowder because it is the closest thing I can think of to medical intervention. My grandfather gets something easy to chew—Salisbury steak? The waiter smiles, writes nothing down, and knows better than to ask if we want a wine list. I want one badly. But Grampa's not popping for booze when there's plenty at home for free. The waiter brings everything exactly right, with a clean, full bottle of Heinz, without being asked. Grampa registers the man's smooth speech and careful manners as a deformity from which one averts the eyes.

The waiter is gay, without a doubt, and when he talks to me, there is a slight shared arch to the eyebrow, the barest of winks. We both know what the old man is, and the value we have in his world. What he would do to us if he knew our full minds. Perhaps wishfully (but as a chubby, smart-mouthed hag from way back, I like to believe it is there), I start to feel that we outnumber the old man. That we are in it. That we are together.

Whatever arrives for Grampa looks like spackle, but he eats with satisfied grunts—the prices are low, much lower than the carrion bird-pecking mark up at all the restaurants at the beach, where only a fool would eat and he's no fool, and that's what matters. He can't taste the stuff anyhow. (When I come back to the Nubble the last time, I will look at the prices on the menus at the beach and feel *exactly* the same way. Feel contempt for the summer people who are foolish enough to pay sucker prices—and no I do not count as a summer person, I am the grand-daughter of a year-rounder, thank you very much. Perhaps it is that contempt that the old man and I have in common? Yuck) I try to swallow the watery, clam-less mess that lands in front of me.

The thought of the drive home is a steady fry to my brain. We could have died a dozen times. And he will never admit that, let alone let me drive home. He would sooner kill me. "Just like Teen."

I make eye contact with my new friend, not in a more-tartar-sauce kind of way, but in a you-cannot-believe-the-day-I-am-having way. He gives me an Oh-girl-of-course-I-could back. And the plan comes fully formed.

The bathrooms are past the till.

"Excuse me for a minute," I say to Grampa, who nods, digs down into his mayo-white coleslaw. I walk over towards the bathroom, stop at the till, lean into my friend, and whisper, like I have been leaning in and whispering to him since puberty, like he is the only thing that got me through grade eight dances, "He's got the keys to my car. I've got to get them away from him. I'm going to pick his pocket on the way back to the table. Can you distract him when you see me go by?"

He accepts the lean-in, accepts the whisper, in a first-slow-dance-of-the-night, arm-around-me-like-he-isn't-actually-hot-for-my brother kind of way.

"Got you."

I bide my time. I want Grampa to be done, but not up, when I get back.

Synchronous with my return, my friend crosses to our table. As he leans down to talk in my grandfather's good ear (he figured that one out in the first five seconds too), I bend to put my purse on the floor beside the old man's coat. Slide my hand into his right pocket. I know it's there because he's right-handed, like everyone in the family except me and Teen. Wrap my fingers around the rental car key.

As a born criminal—moonshiner, safe-cracker, and today, unlicensed driver—my grandfather ought to be proud of this lift, which is clean and soundless.

My friend is leading the old man up to pay, helping him on with his coat, asking gracious questions about the rest of the day. I head straight out. My grandfather doesn't tip to speak of, so, I realize partway to the exit, I should go back and leave everything in my wallet for my friend. But I am fighting for the life of the mother of my children, and I can't risk the detour.

The heavy muffling restaurant doors take their time, but finally open. I bolt out to the car. Jump in, strap in as if that will make it official enough to convince him, and pull up, barring the exit. Throw open the passenger side door.

My now grinning friend ushers my grandfather out the door. The old man stares at the open seat.

"Jump in Grampa."

He hesitates. I am a female, and females do not drive when there is a man. Particularly when there is a bloody-minded, immune-to-the-attacks-of-age-because-he- always-wins, antique buffalo of an American man, waiting to take the wheel. But my friend is now oh so courteously holding the car door for him, offering a hand.

"I'll drive."

"No Grampa. I'm the only one legal in this car." I am afraid he will shout (so what?). I am afraid he will throw a tantrum (and then, so what? I can take him). He is a hard man, and the women in my family have always been afraid of him. But that's fine. I am good at being afraid. And besides, I have my friend.

He can't fight with me about this without betraying his discomfort to the help. He ignores the offered hand and drops heavily into the seat. I throw the car into drive, and look out the window. Lock eyes with my friend, tall, elegant and steady as a lighthouse.

"I will love you forever."

"Oh, you gals always say that."

Mine 2018

And so, past the grey stretch of sand, the white skein of wave, out the point and into the driveway on Driftwood Lane.

Run up the steps to the cottage. My eyes dart. Colour's changed but I knew that from the online photos. The ship's bell hanging by the door is gone, as is the feeding-the-gulls plank that was nailed to the railing. And the bird feed box is full of decorative cushions for an elegant patio set. Still, it is the deck. I look down below and see a patch of lilies growing from the lawn, see my hands and Teen's planting the bulbs, forty-six years before. Look up at the Nubble; feel shy as a long-absent lover. And then to the pond. The big ocean. All of it.

A series of fumbles with a complex, digital lock.

I go in.

The lovely owner has a self-admitted beach-associated decorative item problem. There are aquatic themed gewgaws everywhere. Even the table napkins tell us that "Life's a Beach." I feel oddly short of breath and pace around the rooms, trying to find Teen's house under the Cape Cod kitsch. I focus on the handles of the kitchen cupboards, there since the place was built, scalloped copper grips, beautiful and sturdy and older than me. Mine.

I stand very still. I hear a soft coughing from the back bedroom. Which is nuts and impossible. And so, is nothing that Eric needs to know about.

"Let's go to the rocks."

Eric stares at me. We just got in. Wasn't that the point? Like, the huge big arc of my life point?

"I need to get down to the water."

—

"No trespassing."

We have gone further down the lane and headed for the path that leads to my rock and the water. A voice comes from one of the windows behind us. Fuck. I was sure that house was empty. There hadn't been a sign of life.

"Pardon?" The great Canadian fall back.

"There's no trespassing. This is private land."

I don't know if this is our old neighbour. Or her daughter. She'd be twenty years older than me.

"I beg your pardon. This was my grandparents' place and I —"

"There's no trespassing."

This is the only path to my rock. I have to get there. It's mine. And this old bitch has put up a sign and painted No Trespassing on the only way through to it ... and there's no climbing the boulders between here and Nubble Light Park. Not for me. Not anymore.

After one thick envelope, Gabrielle's miracle, three flights, one rental car, thousands of dollars, this old harridan, who doesn't know me from Adam, is between me and my rock.

"My grandfather put in this path," I scream at the window without a face, "And I have quite possibly life-changing catharsis things I *need* to do down there."

Only of course I don't say that. I'm Canadian now.

We both scuttle away, and Eric says, "Want to get some dinner?"

Sensibly. Rightly. He's clearly in on it with her.

I head for the car.

"Could have been worse," I say, hoping words will calm the roil in my gut, "We could have been brown. She'd'a shot us."[27]

"Maybe just called the police."

"Grampa would'a shot us."

Eric takes me to eat at the restaurant on Long Sands Beach, though we can ill afford it. When it was a 1960s take-out stand, grownups would give you a buck and you could pad down the waterline and shove sandy money over the counter and be given the best fried clams in the world in a red and white striped box, mixed with clam-and-fried fish-flavoured french fries. Smothered in Heinz ketchup. Leaving one hand free for a very cold Pepsi.

But now it's a whole window-on-the-sea deal with waiters who have mid-Atlantic accents and the ability to discuss the wildly overpriced wine list at length. The fried clams are thirty dollars USD. And I can't do it—I decide we'll just go to Short Sands tomorrow and get them take-away, hot and cheap as they should be. I order cioppino, not because I crave fish and broth (I don't, I want my goddamn fried clams), but because it is the cheapest thing on the menu. We eat and watch the sun setting discreetly through the tempered glass. And then we go for a now moonlit stroll along Long Sands.

And I start to breathe, because this beach is still mine. It is unchanged and wonderful and I have walked it a thousand times, head down, checking for intact moon snails and razor back clam shells still hinged into a perfect set of wings.

The following things happen.

I get afraid that I will have to pee (I am always afraid that I will have to pee when I walk because since the third, ten-pound, two foot tall, born-sideways baby, I always have to pee when I walk).

I walk faster, trying to get to the public washroom. No difficulty

---

27. For some reason, talking about guns always brings back my New England accent.

there. I know exactly where it is. But my legs don't seem to know about the no difficulty part. Or maybe they aren't mine anymore. Maybe they belong to a partially crippled woman who has recently had a catastrophic fall, and this grey sliding stuff under her feet is unstable. And they don't do unstable.

I am staggering.

I see a man on the sidewalk above the beach. He is staring as my legs simply fail. Not tire. Not hurt in a way that I can push through. They refuse to be legs, and become something soft and disconnected from me. I grape-vine over the sand. The guy above must think I'm drunk. Eric, ahead of me, turns to see me collapse on a low rock.

I no longer need to pee. That's taken care of.

The Nubble red-winks, but not at me.

"Eric? I don't think I can walk back."

His face gets everything.

"I'll go get the car," and he lopes back, easy as I should be easy, smooth as I should be smooth in this place. My place. My home. I stand, determined to walk up the stairs from the beach to meet him. It is a sand and acid-between-the-legs proposition. Eric helps me into the car, and I do not cry.

Asking 1996

After the lunch, after Grampa slowly climbs up the porch steps and flings himself back into his chair, sets the TV to its highest volume, drowning out the possibility that a girl child just drove him home, after that. I remind Grampa that I'm leaving the next morning.

"I'm worried about you," I say, "You get dizzy on the stairs. A lot. I'm thinking maybe it's time to move somewhere they can take care of you."

He bats my words out of the air. "Not going in. Take everything. It's no good."

"It's your money Grampa—if you want to spend it on care for yourself, you should. We're all up in Canada and we can't come often enough to make sure you`re okay."

"Could I come live up thay'uh with you?"

What the actual fuck?

Take a moment. Look to the Nubble. *Okay,* it says, *you want to be a keeper's daughter? For real?* I have just been offered my opportunity to do what a keeper should do. Slide a peapod boat down that ramp below the boat house and launch into the storm, try to save the wrecked. Reject fear. Stand fast. Be the lighthouse.

Say yes.

So I do. Of course I do. He's a pissing, mean horror show, but everyone knows what you have to do when you have a sick old man alone and howling. If you want to do as keeper's daughter would. As my Auntie Pam did. And, as I should have done, for Teen.

And it is what my mother certainly won't do. And I don't blame her.

After Grampa's gone, when she cleans out this cottage, Mom will search out a paddle, lathed in our centuries-old woodworking shop on Adams Street, smoothed and polished. Nicely ridged grip, fitted to a particular hand by one James A. Adams to more effectively discipline his only daughter. She burns that.

"Marry me kid, and I'll keep you in lollipops," my dad said when he proposed, offering my mother sweets instead harshness, and she took it, took him, and ultimately took us half a continent away, implicitly saying no and goodbye to the stick and the hand that held it.

And when my family went back to Maine for a visit a few years after our move to Canada, Mom made that implicit "no" very explicit.

I am nine. Lying on the bed in Teen's bedroom sleeping off too much sun. Brother Steve, six, cries. He doesn't like the food. I hear Grampa say something about Steve eating what's given him. Steve cries more.

Then the scuff of chairs (Grampa going to hit Steve).

MOM (her own force-feedings in mind, probably—my grandfather cramming hated fish down her throat and then yelling as she vomited it up): "Don't you dare ..."

GRAMPA: "Get him—you get out—"

Screen door slamming. They are leaving the cottage, heading to my Burke cousin's place across the meadow, which my family is renting for the visit.

TEEN: "Oh Jim."

GRAMPA: "Never want to — she can — go to hell ..."

My mother has told her father No. She has put her body between him and her son, and left. Fuck the money. Fuck a lifetime of placation. No one is going to hit her boy.

Which is, in the long, long view, awesome. Fantastic. Except. She's forgotten me. Simply ridden the adrenalin out the door and blanked on the whole existence of another kid.

It takes moment for me to know this. It takes another moment to understand what I have heard, am hearing. Teen's soft crying and "how could yous" and Grampa telling her to shut up.

I get up and choose, very deliberately and calmly, to cry. Arrange my face into tragedy. Fear. Watch myself choose this, too. Walk into the argument like wading into high surf. Use my sobbing to halt the waves.

They both turn and see me standing, face squeezed to guarantee production of tears. It gets very quiet. "Oh God," says Teen, and grabs me. Grabs the car keys. Takes me out of the cottage and into the sun.

Everything is normal and bright again, wild roses scenting everything.

We drive along Nubble Road past the cliffs. We're out of the cottage that has become a clenched fist, and Teen is beside me. The part where I was left behind isn't great but I suspect there will be sweets or something better to ease that bite — though what is better than sweets? — but we're in the white Saab with red leather seats, and we're coasting past the Nubble, and what does Teen keep talking about?

"You know what your grandfather is doing Kelley? Back there? He is crying. He is crying." This is a very disturbing thought and I wish Teen hadn't made me think it. Crying is my thing. Grampa crying would be one of my seven signs of the coming apocalypse, if I knew about the coming apocalypse at this point. "Because he has driven everyone that could love him away. And now he is alone. And so he cries."

I am thinking at this point maybe we should go back. I feel bad that my grandfather is crying alone. But Teen drives me to the cottage where my family is.

I give Mom a good hard look.

"You left me."

"You were fine." Hardly the reaction I was going for. Should I cry again?

"I heard the yelling." Squeeze out a couple of hot ones. Sniff.

"I'm sure you did."

"Oh Ruth, she was so upset," Teen pipes in, and then fades from this memory, so I imagine she was not invited to stay. I was sent to my room, having done something intangibly wrong by being left behind. Having witnessed something private. And bloody.

Teen and Grampa came to visit us in Canada twice after saying of the No but something broke between my mother and her father that day. Something more iron than bone, and jagged.

So maybe he's asking me because he's already tried Mom, and she's said no again? Or maybe he knows better than to try. It doesn't matter. Teen already told me how it will be if I don't take him. He will cry. He will be alone and frightened. That day he drove Mom away, he still had Teen to "Oh Jim" him, and take the brunt of his rage and shame. But he's killed her. And so there's only me for him to ask.

So I do it. And it is a nightmare. Arranging his travel. Closing the cottage. Trying to get him to pay for any of it. Setting Eric and my small house up to accommodate an old man with limited mobility, incontinence, and the emotional discipline of a two-year- old way past naptime who keeps having little strokes.

In fact it takes all of six months and endless wrangling with his lawyer, Immigration Canada, and the IRS man, who is not happy that Mr. Adams wants to move any of his assets out of the country. He comes to our house in the middle of the greyest, coldest, muckiest, not-spring-yet April ever. I settle him in my Tercel two-door held together with duct tape and drive him to my house, which is too small. My cooking is too spicy. We don't eat enough meat. Regina is cold and flat and I only want him here to get his money and I'm getting a surprise because there's none coming my way. My children are spoiled and weak and need discipline, and a couple of times I have to step in. I take in the shock on the kids' faces as they understand what I have stopped, putting my body between them and the old man's raised hand.

I have to call 911 I can't remember how many times, his TIA's get worse from the moment he arrives; he's stressed; he doesn't know where he is and what's going on half the time and it's terrifying for him, meaning he cannot be alone ever. Eric (who I cannot apologize to enough. We weren't doing all that well before Grampa arrived, and I said yes before I talked to Eric, so I am *so* in the wrong) and I hardly speak or touch for most of the time he is with us — it is too weird with the old man sleeping next door. And then it doesn't occur to us. I realize one day that I don't feel married anymore, and I look at Eric. He meets my eyes briefly and looks away. Nope, neither does he.

Getting the old man on and off the toilet is the worst. It's not the shit. I have had babies and wiping asses is nothing. It is how he hates me every time I do it that leaves me shaking. It is how the hate competes with the stink of him in the small bathroom that we have rigged with bars and steps and a raised and cushioned seat that is hell to keep clean. I have to fight the vomit in my throat as I put wet wipe to withered ass, then pull up his pants, the bend putting me face-to-face with his bald and terrible junk. Fight the urge to dodge the fist I can tell he is dying to send my way.

"He's —" I try to talk to my mother about what it. Not to get her to take him. I know that's not on (but dear god, yes, why doesn't she take him?). Just so someone who understands what my grandfather is can bear witness to my days.

"*Now* you know what it's like," says my mom and hangs up.

And it's not much good because he dies on the way to the bathroom, four months after I finally roll him off the plane. I hear the fall, the inelegant meat tumble of a big body whose operating system has lost power all at once. I am trying to get some supper before Eric gets home. (I know well-cooked rice and beans will not make him love me again, but I try nonetheless). Shouting to the dispatcher, who is on the other end of the kitchen phone line, the receiver for which dangles from the wall, I give mouth-to-old-bristly-mouth, count the CPR slam and pumps like I've been taught, and it's doing nothing. He's a wet bag of cement (literally, his pants are dark-stained down the front, and I have to wipe vomit from his mouth before I can try to push air into him), becoming a cold wet bag of cement—and then the flashing lights and the click and roll of the stretcher, and the ripped open plastic husks of huge needle casings and discarded blue gloves everywhere and still he's dead.

(Well. It wasn't hear / shout to dispatch. It was hear/look/stand very still, hang in the moment, breath in the silence / take his pulse, see the lack of breath / think "yes" / shout to dispatch. Etc.)

Eric comes home and sees me sitting crouched on the floor, gathering bits of surgical rubbish. "It's over," I say, and start to cry.

Working on a Memoir 2018

Eric keeps trying. It's Day Three of our trip. As Eric understands it, we have come to York Beach for me to work on a memoir. This is clear, and offers structure and a mission. My complete discombobulation is off-plan and unsettling and can be fixed. And so he tries.

Making arrangements for the artifacts Gabrielle has so carefully saved for us (I fret about going over on our luggage weight limit). Taking me to the York's Wild Kingdom, an amusement park and zoo that I absolutely adored as a child (everything but the merry-go-round is new, and so wrong, and I can't walk long enough to be of any use, and I am hot and ashamed). Taking me to sit on the beach. (I attempt frisking in the surf. The familiar ebb-pull of the sand from under my feet has a new meaning as I fall over. Eric pulls me from the waves). He breaks out his ace. And it has nothing to do with writing, though he may view it as a creative prompt.

His ace is a diamond. But blue. Bitter on the tongue; I know this because I've caught crumbs of it, after Eric crunched his Viagra instead of swallowing, the equivalent of pouring gas into the carburetor to get 'er going. Eight pills to a box. We go through a box every two to three weeks, more on holidays. At least 20 boxes a year. (Not covered by any health plan because sex is not health, it's lifestyle, and my husband's nerve damage could also be addressed by us never having sex again.)

You're doing the math—yes. We have sex at least twice, often four times a week—that's over thirty-eight years. Some weeks it's three times a day. Some months it's not at all. I sat down and figured it out. I've probably had sex with Eric more than 4,000 times. *No way*, you're saying. Sex gets tired. It gets the Seven Year Itch. The Same Old Honey Pot Blues. A hankering for someone who likes pina coladas and getting lost in the rain. Sex settles. Because of the kids. The money. The fear that no one else will take you, now that you have that baby belly/fallen ass/nose hair/sag. Because bodies at rest ... etc. Sex becomes rote with someone you remember fancying once, but not why, and accepts that a resigned life is better than an empty one. Besides you are totally too old.

I don't know. Maybe it's because I'm a very particular sex addict. Despite my medicinal orgasm requirements, the rest of the planet I can take or leave. I start to ache for Eric about three minutes after we make our particular "that's all folks!" noises and fall back sweaty, eyes closed, taking the extra minute before we survey the damage wrought. Maybe it's because we're family in a lot of different ways: husband and wife, mother and father, but also a Peter Pan/Lost Boys sort-of parentless band of two. We found each other living in rabbit pelts, getting good with our slings, and saw an opportunity for something else. Something with a roof on it, smoke and soup steam rising from the chimney. We know the worth of that, use that knowing to prop walls. Steady the stack. Hangs stones from the thatch to stymie windy wolves and pirates.

Or maybe *everyone* is like this and the whole getting tired of the same person thing is a myth perpetuated by capitalism to sell us breath mints.

But staleness and resignation being inevitable is the story that has hung over me every day I've stayed with Eric. I never felt it, but I watched, noted the omens, waited for the moment that Eric did. He would look at me and say it wasn't me, it was him, but, he was taking the money he'd been socking away a little at a time for years so he could go live on a beach in Thailand with her/him/them ... just someone who is NOT all the things I am.[28]

All that considered, when Eric finds me (having spent the day not writing and avoiding the other bedroom down the hall, and the sounds I am definitely not hearing in there) standing mournfully in the closet in my grandfather's bedroom, looking at a set of plain wooden dowels, muttering, "my grandfather built this for his belts. That's real," he pops a blue pill and makes a modest proposal that I am generally inclined to accept. I mean, the longer I can keep him in bed, the longer I can put off his flight to Phuket.

Besides:

1. That he is still asking should be all that matters. (hmmmm)
2. It's amazing how this can totally work from the waist down when the rest of me is in another part of the cottage. (oh)
3. If I could get over the raging sense of failure, I'd be having a really good time (oooh like that there then).
4. It is wasteful to get hung up on the one thing that's off when so much of this is (OOOOH! Blimey!) good.

And then I hear it again, a small, sawing pull of air and cough, coming from down the hall. I close my eyes tighter still and simply hold on.

---

28. Yes, there are many variants of the how-Eric-will-leave-me fantasy. There are no versions where he stays.

Asking 2 1996

Grampa asks me after I come back from rock-climbing.

I'm not as good as when I climbed at eighteen. At thirty-four, I've had two of my three babies and the arthritis that will finally cripple me is already a presence and I am afraid on the rocks for the first time ever. Still. Foot propped here. Hand pushed there. Look and see the next point. Know without knowing the angle to shift hip and lunge. The step that will hold. The step that will break. My heart sings a little. I can still do it.

I'm wearing my trench coat—a ridiculous caped over-priced thing that a saleswoman hustled me into, assuring me that it flattered my spreading form. "It's very fashion forward." She leans in to keep it our secret. "Fashion forward" means something that will be regretted moments after purchase, and makes me look like a 1930s closet-case super villain. It is inappropriate. But I have nothing else waterproof with me and the sky is heavy and warning.

Teen is rumbling at me again. She wants to know what I was thinking. After escaping death on the rocks at the Nubble last night, I am climbing again? With rain coming?

"*Oh Kelley. Take my hand. Take my hand now. This isn't good, honey.*" My frantic ghost.

I shake her off. What the hell. If I ruin the coat, I won't have to think about how much it cost, and how little I like it. Keep going. With nursing the second baby came carpal tunnel damage to my hands and I'm feeling its nervy needles every time I slap my palms to rough stone. Who cares? I belong here. I was taken away and told to forget so I remembered harder. I am the rock-climbing, sea-loving, not yet a keeper's daughter (but I haven't given up). And I am smart. And I am pretty. Teen was a batty old pill and booze lover who is still driving me crazy, but that's what she said—and here, now, at the lighthouse, on the rocks, I believe her.

I taste salt on my lips. Squint, measure the rise in the tide.

"It's okay Teen. I've got this."

"Oh look Kelley. Look. You can see Boone so clearly. That's where they ate the carpenter."

"Yes. I remember," looking out to the further, lonely lighthouse on Boone Island, the site of Teen's favourite wreck and cannibalism story. We don't need to go over it again. "Sea's like glass today. We'll go to the beach when I get back, okay? I'll get a poking stick."

I make it back without falling to my death, which pleases Teen. Doesn't stop her fussing, as I pick my way back up the path. *"You must use the rubbing alcohol as soon as you get back to the house, Kelley. See there. Poison ivy. Three leaves. They turn rusty red in the fall."*

So I rub my legs down—I don't think it does anything but make me smell like a thermometer, but at least she can calm down. Pour myself a bourbon and ginger without being offered, and go to sit in the dark living room with Grampa. I remind him that I'm leaving the next day.

"Grampa, I'm worried about you," I say, "You get dizzy on the stairs. A lot. I'm thinking maybe it's time to move somewhere they can take care of you."

He bats my words out of the air. "Not going in. Take everything. It's no good."

"It's your money Grampa—if you want to spend it on care for yourself, you should. We're all up in Canada. It's too far away for us to make sure you're okay."

"Could I come up thay'uh and live with you?"

What the actual fuck?

"*Oh Kelley. Stay off the black rocks.*"

I am reaching for Teen's hand.

I look at him. I walk over and open a blind, look at the Nubble. Teen continues her warning. *Not safe. Not safe.* She is all but flashing a red light, and her voice is pitched to the Nubble's horn.

Is he kidding? *He killed her.* Not because he wanted her dead. On the contrary, he hates her being dead. He killed her because he was too *scared* of being the stupid chump who gets soaked by a hospital where aspirin costs more than steak. He let Teen drown in her own lungs so he wouldn't feel ... that. And now he wants me to —

I think I am thinking this. In fact I am shouting this. I am shouting like my mom did when he came at Steve. I am shouting like him.

I am afraid of him. It is burned into my DNA, this fear, specific and gendered and national and absolute, along with, but different than, the anxiety that eats a little more of my lifespan every day. But the daughter of Ruth Adams, who was the daughter of Jim Adams, knows how to respond to specific, targeted fear.

Hit it. Hit it hard.

"If you didn't want to be alone, you shouldn't have driven away everyone who could love you except her. Not if you couldn't be bothered to keep her alive. Now you will cry. *Cry.*" She gives me the words, my Teen, my lighthouse, my pill-popping, drunk-by-lunch-but-still-as-trustworthy-as-anything-in-my-world warning of sunken danger.

He is shouting now too, I don't hear what because the roar of blood surf in my ears is drowning it all and I want to run. Where? Her room? No it doesn't lock and he'll kill me too. There may still be guns. There are certainly hundreds of razor sharp knives—he hones every blade in the house obsessively—there's a pair of sewing shears that ought to be registered with the police. I back to the door, grab my purse, and push the screen door open. Go out on the porch, and throw up my arms.

Hear the answer, coming from the point of the Nubble. It hasn't been too long —they remember the arms thrown up in the air. The day old bread hitting the shingles. They remember her. They think I am her, and they come, as a squadron, squawking and murmuring and hovering and hopping, dozens of gulls, her gulls. I stand in the room of their sound and know he cannot touch me.

We are so happy here.

"I know, Teen."

He stands staring out at me in the sun. The gulls all around me seem to be something he can't quite sort.

"Ruth—Teen—Kelley— you, you ... don't—?" his words chug out like a one-lunger engine's sputter.

The gold of his wire glasses glints in the light that's broken through. His eyes are gone, the lenses discs of ocean glinting. I take a step back. I see him start to lose me in the sun ... as a few more gulls fly up, and start to scold, bread promised but undelivered.

And then I am gone—and take her with me.

Wreck 2018

We have sex. Lots and lots of sex. In my grandfather's room, not in his actual bed, that's long gone, but still. Being in that bedroom requires a certain amount of cognitive dissonance right there. We do what we do whenever we get away from our life and have time alone. Like this is any other cottage. Like this isn't the most important cottage. Like everything in my life is not resting on the knife edge of these four days. Like I can't hear the cough. We get out the magic pills and have lots and lots of sex.

And it doesn't work. For pretty much the first time, it doesn't work.

Drag my sticky self to the porch, and my laptop. Click away about my rocks, my cottage, my beach, my, my, my. Look over to the lighthouse, bright and cheery in the sun, wearing scaffolding. People who *are* allowed on the island, who have real reasons to be there, are giving the lamp tower a fresh coat of paint. I am a tourist watching that happen. This whole journey to find my safe place, my home, my peace, and somehow hold onto it, is shit I just made up, I tell the cough, even though there is no cough, no dead grandmother haunting, nothing but my own single-minded, and uniquely narcissistic inflation of some garden-variety home-sickness. I am missing the point. I force my eyes back to the lighthouse.

"What do you want to do?" Eric calls from the bedroom.

Twitch. No idea. My urgent need to get here has turned to paralysis.

I'm supposed to be doing *something*. I'm supposed to be finding the end to this. A way out of this mess. The whole of everything that I have longed for my entire life is available to me, and I do not know how to be with it. The house, Gabrielle's house, is lovely and quaint and comfortable and thoughtful and God is good, Gabrielle, and blesses you in your new home, but it is not doing what I thought it would do.

I have gotten here. I have gone in. I feel.

Nothing. (Liar)

I feel panic. (Duh)

I feel I am failing, and I should die. (And I *still* haven't gone in her room, says no one in particular and I certainly don't hear it, because it's a METAPHOR! My big aha! moment on the car ride here was not supposed to lead to an actual haunting. I glare at the Nubble like it's holding out on me.)

I edit the same six paragraphs I've been trying to get right for an hour. Realize that I am staring at the computer screen like Grampa stared at the TV, and the light house is RIGHT THERE, and I'm not even looking at it.

My back hurts. I make myself go in, grab a pillow from anywhere but her bed. This is silly. I was in there after she died. I went through her things, stole her jewelry.

"What do you want to do?" Eric asks again, looking out to the sea and the road and all the things that are not me sitting hunched and rancid on the deck, where the bell, the board, and my grandmother should be.

"Nothing? I don't know."

I can't get to my rocks. I can't find a batch of fried clams that I don't have to pawn an organ to buy. I can't find the ending to my "healing journey." I thought if I was in this place, this wonderful place, the harm and hurt and crazy would all melt away, but the part of my odd brain that just refuses to process certain things has pulled a fast one on me yet again. I have come to make everything better *to the house where he killed her.* Hands up, who figured that out way before me? Who has been asking all along: *Does she even remember that? Does she even understand that she is waxing rhapsodic about going home to a crime scene?* Who does that? Who packs a bag and says, hey, let's go get our beach on, in a place where something *completely traumatic* happened?

Talk about shit I just made up. I wasn't born here. I didn't grow here. I don't sound like anyone who did, and the noise I make about being from the coast, and knowing the tides, and "being out the boats" is a sentimental pastiche of thread memory and outright fiction that I have built *over top* of what really happened here as some kind of add-water panacea for problems that I do not want to address. *If I could only be at the lighthouse. If I could only stay by the sea.* My lying would stop. My rat-gnawed heart would slow. I would be well. Instead I have simply been handed a memo—"Do *something* about your dead-two-decades grandmother. And stop bothering me."

My goodness that is all a sloppy bit of curation. A lie that I have used to deceive a chump. The chump being me.

Look for something to save me in the items Gabrielle found in the attic and left for us. Silver spoons. Fabulous hats. Many maps. All in a wooden chest hand-made by my great-grandfather Frank—we'll have to leave that with Pam—it's not carry-on. And Grampa's photo album from 1923.

And there he is young and landed and full of his own promise. There are his chums and girlfriends, hiking Mt. Wachusetts, and boating on the family lake. And there is Teen, showing up part way through the year, a beauty with high cheekbones, long rippling brown hair that kinks at the exactly the same spot behind the left ear as mine. A healthy, gorgeous gal, a jazz baby, who made her own money, and had a choice between juicy sin in New York or marriage with James A. Adams, of the Westminster Adams. And when James A. drove his buggy up to the train station where she waited, portmanteau in hand, ready to leave decency behind, and shouted, "Teen, stop being stupid. Get in, and marry me," she *did*. She chose a life, whole and complicated, well before I ever met her. And I will never understand it. I'm not supposed to. It's not my business.

The only business I have here is in the second bedroom that I apparently haven't got the moral fibre to enter, and besides why should I? There is no fixing that.

I look back to the view. The sun glimmers off the ocean as it promised. The lighthouse takes my gaze, being only what it is, and wonders what I want that it's not. "I am so tired of you." I say out loud to myself. But the lighthouse hears it. And shuts its face to me.

I see the change. It is just a lighthouse. Whoever it was before has given up on me and moved on.

Asking 3 1996

My grandfather asks, my last day in Maine, as I sit on the edge of the sofa, rental keys in hand, ready to drive to Logan. I start to say what I have come to say.

"Grampa, I'm worried about you," I say, "You get dizzy on the stairs. A lot. I'm thinking maybe it's time to move to somewhere — "

He bats my words out of the air. "Not going in. Those places ... take everything. It's no good."

"It's your money Grampa — if you want to spend it on care for yourself, you should. We`re all up in Canada. It's too far away for us to make sure you're okay."

"Could I come up thay'uh and live with you?"

What the actual fuck?

I say as little as possible of course.

It's not that I don't know he shouldn't be here alone. It's not that I can't forgive him for killing Teen. It's not even that my life is now Canada. Not my home, but my life. My children are Canadian. My husband. Our family lives in a Canadian way. We say sorry to the babies as they emerge from my womb, sorry for the inconvenience, and we mean it. We have less money, and more kindness. We are not Ad(d)ams. We are not even more than half Burkes. So yes, I don't want his alien rancor and meanness anywhere near what we have built. Like I *really* don't. But it's not that.

Aunty Pam knows what the answer should be. My angry mother, made by this angry man, would have another theory. The lighthouse (which I can't see behind Grampa's thick dusty blinds) knows the answer too, for anyone with any claim to being a keeper's daughter. But mostly I know what Teen *can't* answer, because, when I knew that she wasn't safe here, I didn't take her to live with me. What she can't say is that this is my opportunity, not to make amends, because throwing whales in the sea be-damned, you can't make amends to the dead, but you can take your punishment. And this is it.

And still. I don't want to do it.

Getting him to Canada would be a nightmare. My house is too small, and I am poor, and shifting the money will be impossible. My mother will hate that I have brought him anywhere near her, and my mom hating scares me (and shames me for being scared). I am not good enough for this. I am not brave enough for this. I am too much of a mess.

I don't want to.

"Grampa, I don't think you would like it where I live. It's very far. And very, very cold in the winter. And they would make you leave all your guns ..."

"Oh."

"My house isn't set up for you. We might have to get you into a retirement home up there anyway."

He looks at me. Calculates what it would mean for me to be able to put him away.

"That might not be so good then."

When I get home and tell Eric what he asked and what I said, he gives me an out.

"If Teen asked, if she'd been willing to leave your grandfather, you'd have said yes. If my aunt needed to stay with us, or yours, we wouldn't think twice. He is who he is. And who he is put him where he is. "

I stare at Eric and nod, not because I know what he is saying is true, but because I wish it was.

I am no keeper's daughter. I had one last chance. Not to make it right. Making it right is lying cold and dead in Mount Pleasant Cemetery, Westminster, Mass. But doing something. Doing the least I could do for her. And I didn't do that.

A few months later, Grampa falls down the cellar stairs. Dead. Maybe a little stroke? I never know whether it's that or the fall. It is November, and the Massachusetts ground too frozen to take him. Months after, in the middle of a separate conversation, Mom mentions that people she knows back in Westminster were out walking their dog past the cemetery and saw the back hoe finishing a dig. Asked. It was his box going in. Couldn't stay to watch, the morning was cool and they had to keep moving. Thought Mom would want to know.

I start to cry.

"Oh please," says Mom, cutting the call short.

I will never really be at the lighthouse again.

Westminster, Stupid 2018

Upstate Massachusetts in June is nothing but cloying, industrial smoke-scented humidity. I hate heat. It doesn't make me faint, it makes me stabby. Very stabby. Usually, by a hot day's end, I owe apologies to Eric, the kids, the dogs, the neighbours, people in cars, people out of cars. And squirrels. Squirrels are bastards.

Right now there's only Eric.

After four days, we have left the cottage. Left a gift for Gabrielle, one of Teen's whale figurines. And a thank you note for everything. Like it's okay.

Eric takes me to Westminster. To Teens' grave.

"We can go to the store. Get some steel wool to clean the lichen off the headstone. We can bring flowers and plant them."

"With what?"

"We can buy a trowel."

"A trowel?"

"Yes."

"And then what? Throw it away?"

"That woman, where we're staying. She'll have something we can borrow. At least let's clean the stone."

He thinks Teen is here. Under this rock. Lying in a ridiculously expensive box under badly kept grass, settling into bones and tufts of hair. Idiot. She's in the back bedroom at the cottage. Where I abandoned her. Again. My brain is not working and my mouth tastes of bitter and piss.

He wants to do this one thing, scrape a little moss off a stone that says ADAMS, on the back side of which she is listed as Ernestine E. Brewer Adams (1906-1995), above my grandfather and to the left of his grandparents, Aldin and Lizey Anne, and his parents, Jessie and Frank. I want to get the hell out. I hate it. Hate that the stone says she is here. Hate that this Adams ground believes it can eat her. I hate.

"It's a big piece of granite standing in the rain in Massachusetts. There'll be lichen again in a week."

Eric's expression goes blank. Zero affect. It is his version of kicking dirt in my face.

"Whatever. She's your grandmother."

"I don't know why we're here."

"I *thought* you were writing a memoir."

Was he always this stupid?

We've been to Adams Street. The old houses are heritage sites and so very little has changed. As we poke around my former home, which is nicely kept and discretely added to, a man comes out to greet/challenge us.

"Can I help you?"

"Sorry. I was born here. This was ... my house."

A pause. He looks at me hard.

"You must be an Adams." I nod. And he nods back, which for Massachusetts is a big sloppy kiss. Does not invite us in.

We've been to my old library—I know the way there without question. The entire building that I knew is now the entrance, but it smells the same. We go to a rummage sale at the First Congregational Church, where I get a member's discount, even though I haven't attended since 1972. I've even hovered reluctantly, later in the afternoon, as Eric visits the Westminster Historical Society (as an amateur genealogist, he has an uncomfortably intimate relationship with this august body). The musty room is a bake oven, and my muscles are locked in run-away readiness. But I discover that the old man sitting in it, logging images on an ancient computer, is in fact a child I knew more than half a century ago. He holds out a photo of a large group of young people for identification and says, "We thought maybe this was your great-grandmother Jessie" and I look for one second and say "Nope. That's her" pointing to a stunning young woman with the hooded eyes of a hunting bird. Pride flickers briefly through the sultry air; clearly I am still enough of an Adams to know one.

I slap pride away. All I am allowed to feel is the heat and the stupid and the went-to-the-cottage-and-wasted-everything *hate* of it all. This place isn't the lighthouse and so it doesn't count, screw the street I know, rock, tree, and church and all that's not part of the peace that passeth understanding. This is Westminster. This is part of *the rest*. The crazy and sad and drunk, the raised hand, and the lying mouth and the set jaw. I've never needed this. Except, as it turns out, I've never needed the lighthouse either. I made that up.

Only I want to go back and try again because without the lighthouse I don't have anything.

When we get back to the even hotter, making-me-stabbier BnB, Eric walks to the small spare bed in the corner. Jaw set. Drops down and into the fetal position. Boom. Out. Before he gets his second sandal off. Sleep as deep as death.

I look at his curled-from-me back. He has been so good. Driving me about, day after day, as I became increasingly ass-over-tea-kettle, not knowing which way was up, swimming only to find bottom, crazy. And furious—at him. Because he doesn't seem to understand that everything is wrong, everything is lost, and what's more, it always was.

I sit and watch him sleep. Eyes locked. Blink and he will definitely disappear. This time he hates me. His love is now the only thing I will ever have to keep the rats and bats in my belfry at bay, and right here, right now, I've completely lost that. As I have lost the light-house. Or rather, as I never had them, the love or the light, because they are just shit I made up. The tears that were pouring from me twelve hours before (I do not, at this point, remember why I was crying twelve hours before, but I can feel that my eyes have done quite a bit of crying recently) begin again.

Sit more. Thirty minutes more. Forty. Watching him. Breathing salty grief.

Cross to the little bed, and touch his arms. Goodbye.

Am stunned when the arms open. And close. Like the eye of the lighthouse. But around me.

And then, I remember what happened before we left the Nubble.

At the Lighthouse

It is twelve hours before. Our last morning in the cottage. We will go to Westminster next. We are standing in my grandfather's bedroom. I look out the little window in the nook Grampa gave himself when he winterized the cottage. See the sea he came to loathe shining most brilliantly. Loathe it too.

"I've dragged you all this way. And I can't feel it. I can't feel anything. I can't do anything. I can't even walk on the beach. You have done everything for me. And I have given you all these awful days."

"I haven't had awful days." Eric says.

"You haven't had good ones."

"Every day with you is a good day."

I wait for the punchline.

I wait for the punchline.

I wait.

And then I consider. What it might mean if that were true. If after wrecking everything, again. Failing, again. Failing to be smart. Or brave. Or ... anything other than unforgivable. What would it mean if he kept loving me? If I was completely wrong about that—as *well* as everything else?

Walk over. Let him hold me as if he's not a grenade about to go off.

Close my eyes. And breathe.

"*Every* day I spend with you is a good day," he says again.

Look up. "I'll be with you in a minute." And then I walk across the hall and stand in front of Teen's door. Go in.

Tiny room. Serviceable. No window nook built for Teen. Just small high windows. She kept a step stool to look out, and all she could see was Nubble Road with its speeding cars that made her breath come in gulps. Traffic noise drowns out the sounds of the sea.

Bed, chest of drawers brought from Westminster, all gone now. But my hand moves over the chest top that is not there. Over the clothes not hanging in their exact order and size in her closet. Over the hooked loops of her long-gone candlewick spread.

I hear her cough, clearly now, low and rasping ... the strain of it pinning her to the mattress. Her usual scent of soap and dry leaves made over-ripe by fever. Hear my grandfather's step behind me as he says ... what? What could he say, having done this? Even "Do you need anything?" would have been an admission that he made a mistake. So no. Not even that. Just stand. Stare. Stump back to his chair, his blinded windows.

And my Teen is ... scared. She is dying rat-scared. Or so disoriented that there is only confusion and the heat of her body and the wet of her lungs, the tide roaring in and surging down her windpipe. How long? I was told she was dead four hours after he rolled her out of the ambulance and bumped up the porch stairs, dropping her into this dark room. But how long did it take him to come back? Look in again at what was clearly not a mistake and not his fault and discover that she was not breathing? Or not going to breathe much more?

I put my hand on the body not on the bed. After all my protestations, my proclaimed longing, I didn't stop him. I didn't save her. I didn't even save him when he asked. I didn't do a good goddamn thing. I stayed with the family plan of pretending I had no obligations to the world left behind, not because I was a child and didn't know better, not anymore, but because I was an adult, and did know better, but managed to overlook that. I let them all die alone. Let her, who was never perfect, but also never offered me anything but true love, die alone.

"I'm sorry." I say. "I'm sorry." Gulping, shaking, over and over, until the words are less word and more water and wind ... and wait. Wait for her to tell me what the terrified and the slug-shocked know. That what is done can never be undone. That everything that was, is gone. That I cannot be at the lighthouse, not really, not ever. Stupid.

(But what if?)

I feel her reach out. Take my hand. Say something else.

Oh honey. You are so precious.

What?

Get your bucket and pail, Kelley. Get a towel. Off to the beach, we will go. Brum brum brum.

Each *brum* like we're a brass band of two, Teen and I leave the room where nothing can be undone. Skip a little as we make our way to the Saab. Coast down Nubble Road to Long Sands (wheeee!). Park, put five thin dimes in the meter. Take bucket and shovel to the sand. And start to do what can be done.

We *build* a lighthouse. We build it from:

My rock.

My gull.

My big ocean pounding a steady message through the sand: *Welcome keeper's daughter.*

We build it from Eric's hand. Eric's chest. Eric.

My grandmother's face, lined with terror and love.

My grandfather's arms, tying me safe in a storm.

My standing in the living room in Winnipeg with my brother alive, Stevie-grinning, and Jess. Simon & Garfunkel singing "Kodachrome" live in Central Park from the turntable and we're dancing. Mom walks in, joins us. Dad comes home, time bomb in his head not blowing up but beating in its shell, making him ache and mourn. We spin around him. Sing. "*Kodachro-o-ome ... give us those nice bright colors. They give us the greens of summers. Makes you think all the world's a sunny day, oh yeah...*" Laugh. Until Dad does too.

Telling the man from Africa the truth, instead of lying. And him still giving me his smile.

Inviting the Rat of my crazy to tea, (we have crumpets and cheese).

Wrapping around dead Steve's body, so cold and eyeless in the dark. He curls to the warmth of my belly.

Whispering to my finally dying dad, "It's okay. You can be done now."

Going into the room. When it mattered. Wetting Teen's handkerchief with lavender water, laying it on her forehead, fever steaming the scent. I should be calling the ambulance back, telling them to ignore the frightened old man. But this is as much as I can manage. Cooling her face, holding her hands, seeing how my fingers, old now like the rest of me, are hers, down to the whorls of the knuckles. Whispering, "It's okay. Feel that? Little hand in big hand. Hold tight. *You* are so precious, honey."

We poke and dig. Draw water and pack. Of course it won't hold. It's not supposed to. It's made of sand. And memory. And fiction. From forgiveness. And not. Lies. And not. From my kids. My uncle and aunt. My cousins, all Ballerina Pink and Princess Blue of them. The Adams. The Addams. The Burkes.

I use all of it to build a platonic ideal of a house, and a white cylinder capped with a black bowler. Plain. Sturdy as a Greek column. Held by the sea. As trustworthy as anything in the world.

And know it will all be washed away.

"And then honey, we will make another."

For the great lamp's light, I add my standing on the rocks, in the dark, throwing the pilot whale in. I am about to fall into black pain and regret, but who cares? The last whale hits the water. I hear the slap of its tail, the rush of its sweeping up, curving down, and under. I hear *all* Teen's whales find the sea. And the lighthouse's red eye follows her as she, unafraid, finds the sea with them.

"We are so happy here."

I look at the lighthouse. Built on sand, not rock. Like me.

I'm not afraid now either, but I will be, and soon. I will forget, and mis-remember and panic and despair. I will get it wrong and make shit up. But this has happened, and perhaps, I will be able to remember it often enough that it will become part of my curation, part of my truth.

For now, I close my eyes and breathe. Like breathing's something I can do any day of the week.

And it is very very good.

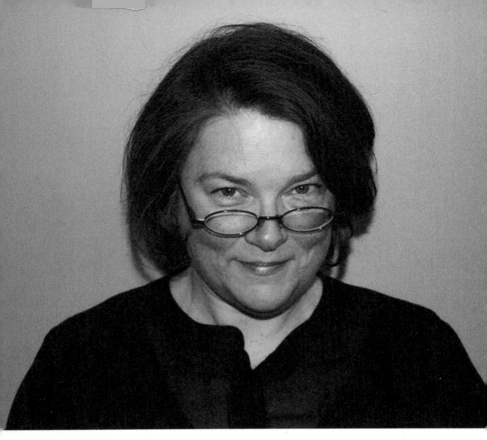

Kelley Jo Burke an award-winning Regina playwright, creative nonfiction writer and documentarian, a professor of theatre and creative writing, and past host of CBC Radio's SoundXchange. She is the 2017 winner (with composer Jeffery Straker) of the Playwright Guild of Canada's national Best New Musical Award for *Us*, which premiered at the Globe Theatre in 2018. Recent plays include *The Lucky Ones*, *The Selkie Wife*, and *Ducks on the Moon*. Her published work includes four books, inclusion in four collections, many periodicals, and she is the creator of eight creative nonfiction documentaries for CBC's IDEAS. She was the 2009 winner of the Saskatchewan Lieutenant-Governor's Award for Leadership in the Arts, the recipient of the 2008 Saskatoon and Area Theatre Award for Playwriting, and has won the City of Regina Writing Award three times. Kelley Jo lives in Regina, Saskatchewan.